COVER UP

TAKING *THE* LID OFF *THE* COSMETICS INDUSTRY

CW01019316

COVER UP

TAKING THE LID OFF THE COSMETICS INDUSTRY

PENNY CHORLTON

To Sue & Graham
& the girls,
with lots of
love from
Pen xx

GRAPEVINE

First published 1988

Illustrations by Ian Dicks

British Library Cataloguing in Publication Data

Chorlton, Penny
  Cover-up: taking the lid off the cosmetics
  industry.
  1. Cosmetics, perfumes & toiletries
  industries
  I. Title
  338.4'76685

ISBN 0-7225-1398-4

Grapevine is an imprint of the Thorsons Publishing Group, Wellingborough, Northamptonshire NN8 2RQ England.

Printed in Great Britain by
Mackays of Chatham, Kent
Typeset by MJL Typesetting Services,
Hitchin, Hertfordshire.

10 9 8 7 6 5 4 3 2 1

CONTENTS

ACKNOWLEDGEMENTS

I'd like to be able to thank the cosmetics industry for their help in researching this book, but alas, I cannot. Not surprisingly, perhaps, none of them wanted to 'get involved' when they heard this was to be a 'consumer' book.

After a less than friendly response to my initial approaches, I discovered that the best I could hope for were company statements in response to nasty or peculiar things I managed to unearth about particular products. Most companies did not even bother to reply — those that did merely put me on their press list which meant endless expensively produced glossy advertising brochures about new products.

My thanks therefore go to Andrew Mayer, my researcher on the *Washington Post,* who delved deep into the files, and, thanks to the accessibility of information in America, provided a great deal of the material on which this book is based.

My sincere thanks, too, to Morton Mintz, investigative award-winning reporter on the *Post* for his constant supply of ideas, information and above all, inspiration.

Finally, thanks to Mitch, my patient husband and professional business partner, for not only putting up with me hogging the study, computer, filing cabinets and bookshelves for two years, but also for his comprehensive support, without which this book most certainly would not have been written.

Dedication
To Mitch, of course, and to my son Jack,
whose conception, gestation and birth
coincided — not always with the greatest
convenience — with the production of
this book.

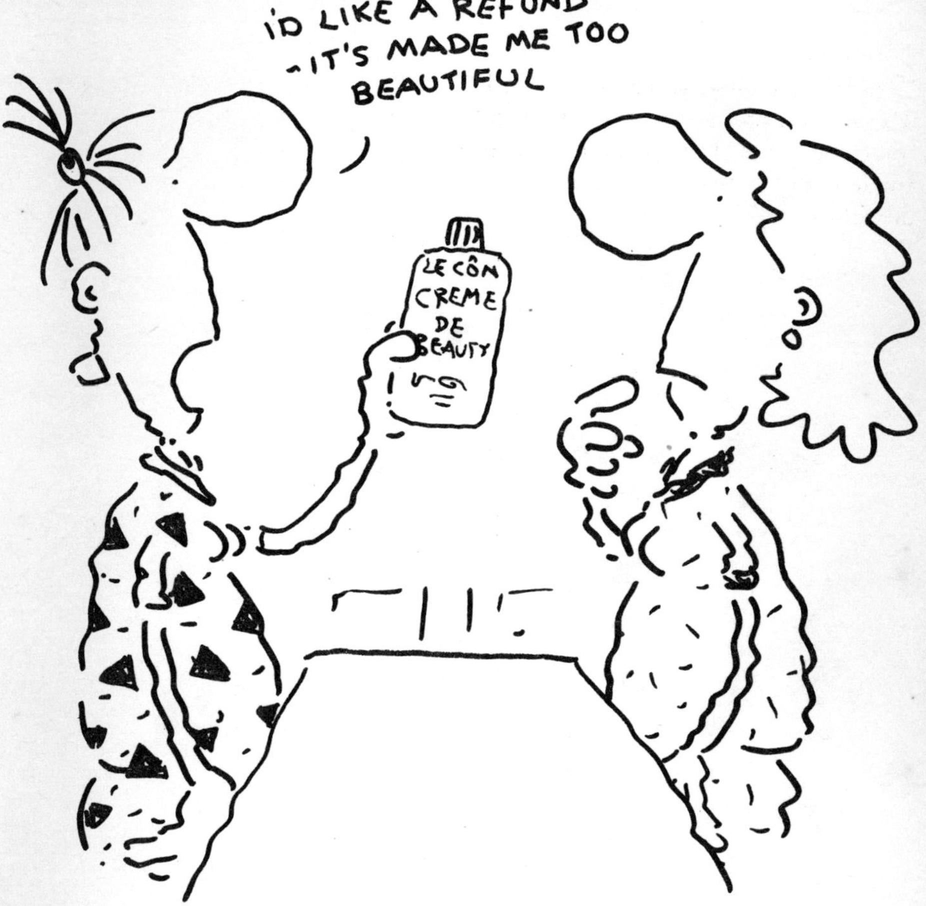
I'D LIKE A REFUND -IT'S MADE ME TOO BEAUTIFUL
LE CÔN CREME DE BEAUTY

INTRODUCTION

This is not another 'how to' beauty book. There are dozens of those, with secret tips from the world's beauties on how you too can look like them — ha ha! What those books don't tell you is what the cosmetics and beauty industry is *about* — what the products contain, why we buy them and whether they work.

The cosmetics industry, which so successfully exploits our insecurities, is not tackled by the consumer organizations. There is no Cosmetics Commission, hardly any Consumers' Association investigations or *Which*? reports, and very little outside interference from government departments. A Department of Trade spokeswoman says that there are two full-time people directly responsible for all national monitoring of the cosmetics, toiletries, and perfumes sold in the UK. In the last two years, the Department issued only three press statements on action taken in this area.

The industry is vast and it touches all of us because we all use cosmetics and toiletries to some extent, every day of our lives, yet, unlike the industries producing food or medical pharmaceuticals, the cosmetics industry is a secret world, a world we know only by the hype, image and impression fed to us by the glossy world of advertising. We use the products of this vast industry because we have been influenced by fashion and habit into believing them to be necessary to our way of living. Are they necessary? Are they *all* necessary?

'In the factory we make cosmetics; in the drugstores we sell hope,' said the late Charles Revson, founder of one of the world's largest cosmetics companies, Revlon. His great rival, the late Elizabeth Arden, once described the cosmetic's industry as 'the nastiest business in the world'.

But although some of us realize we are only buying dreams, most of us, most of the time, expect value for money: products which will do what they claim, with no nasty side-effects.

CONFIDENCE AND KNOWLEDGE

This is not a book which will tell you that all cosmetics are a waste of money — it's more a guide as to what exactly these cosmetics are, why we use them, and why perhaps some of them are a waste of money and even downright harmful, either to ourselves as individuals or to society as a whole.

After reading this book, I don't expect you to clear out your bathroom cabinets and dressing tables and dismiss all cosmetics as rubbish but I *do* hope that you will feel more confident and knowledgeable about the subject in general and about the forces, such as the beauty press, which pressure us into spending a massive £1,500 million a year on creams and potions designed to enhance our appearance.

As I shall show — especially in the chapters on skincare — all cosmetics are basically very similar. Indeed, some formulations are identical, and are made in the same cosmetic laboratories.

The difference, of course, is in the packaging, which often costs more than the ingredients, and, inevitably, in the marketing. Is there any point in paying more than £1.50 for a jar of moisturizer, and are those £75 pots truly capable of working miracles and stripping away those crow's feet and bags from under your eyes?

Of course, part of the fun — and therapy — of using cosmetics and toiletries is the transient feeling of indulgence that we get from buying them and wearing them. Indeed, 50 per cent of all our cosmetics purchases are impulse buys. The 'lift' we get from buying and using these things should not be under-estimated, but the psychology of why and how we decorate ourselves is worth thinking about. You may even find you've been unintentionally arousing all the wrong reactions in the people you've been trying to impress, never mind seduce!

It is easy to deride the heavily made-up sales women and to sneer at women who rely on cosmetics and perfumes as an essential 'prop'. They make easy targets for women who scorn those less confident than themselves who need artifice to bolster their self-esteem.

However, even the most successful of 'superwomen' will check that her hair is in order before going into her executive meeting. And the indomitable Mrs Thatcher, for all her tough no-nonsense image, makes no secret of the fact that she cares very much about her appearance, including her clothes, her hairstyle and her make-up.

Although the title of this book suggests an exposé (and I hope there are some interesting revelations). I don't wish to knock the industry entirely — the world would be a less colourful place without it. I just want to query some of its excesses and practices and to try to sort out the factual wheat from the promotional chaff.

The cosmetics industry constantly comes up with new fads designed to make us throw away last year's unfinished products and buy new ones. Seaweed, mud, and exotic plant species like jojoba and aloe vera have all had their day and 'natural' products are still enjoying enormous popularity because they are supposed to be superior to 'synthetic' alternatives.

'NATURAL' DOESN'T MEAN 'SIMPLE'

Natural products can be very complicated; geranium, for example, has thirty different chemical ingredients which change according to the season and climate. Even the humble cucumber has a long list of ingredients which would make it very hard to reproduce in a test-tube. Yet, because we are presented with 'pure' images, we believe the products to be simple and therefore somehow superior. This may not necessarily be the case. Generally speaking, the more complicated the contents of a product are, the more likely it is to bring us out in spots.

We fall for these 'fads' partly because of what we read in the ecstatic features welcoming their 'discovery' on the beauty pages of magazines, particularly womens' magazines but, as I'll reveal in the chapter on advertising, beauty editors are rarely able to write freely about cosmetics. Their copy is often 'advertorial', which means either that the editorial copy is insisted upon as condition of the placement of lucrative advertisements elsewhere in the magazine, or that future earnings from this essential source must on no account be threatened by critical or hostile prose.

It is significant that when the publishers of this book approached several of the leading women's magazines to see if they would be interested in co-operating in a survey of their readers' use of cosmetics and the hair and beauty industry, the general response was guarded, and in the end most said they would not dare, in case the results offended their advertisers on whom they depended for a large percentage of their income.

THE INDUSTRY NO-ONE CRITICIZES

The cosmetics industry is unique in this, for the media rarely shirk from criticizing other material goods and services, from cars to holidays to restaurants, films, plays, and even, to a lesser extent, fashion, which is a close relative of the cosmetics and perfume industry.

> 'Cosmetic companies have a licence to say whatever they like because no-one has the power, right or inclination to disprove their claims.' *Dermatologist.*

Unfortunately, independent, unbiased advice is not available in the shops either, for retailers have their profits and commissions to think about. Even if they put these considerations aside, they are not qualified to interpret the pseudo-scientific jargon which is employed these days to sell many cosmetics, especially the more expensive skincare lines.

Indeed, even the cosmetic companies are hard-pressed to analyse the claims made by their rivals. Although companies wax lyrical about the scientific 'trials' they have done on their products and the 'astonishing results' they have produced, — do not be misled! For, cosmetics, unlike drugs, do not have to *prove* their effectiveness to any regulatory body. As one leading dermatologist told me, 'Cosmetics companies have a licence to say whatever they like because no-one has the power, right or inclination to disprove their claims.'

LACK OF CONSUMER PROTECTION

In April 1987, the Australian Consumers' Association produced a major report for the country's National Health and Medical Research Council, *Cosmetics Advertising in Australia: The Lack of Consumer Protection.*

The report noted numerous unsubstantiated claims made by many of the leading cosmetics companies, particularly in relation to ingredients such as collagen, elastin, vitamins, fruits, vegetables, herbs, and flowers.

Although, unlike British authorities, the Australian authorities are in the process of introducing partial labelling of ingredients in cosmetics, the ACA concluded:

Serious concerns remain in connection with the misleading nature of many cosmetics advertisements, the lack of useful information available to consumers and the inadequacy of warnings on products . . . This is particularly worrying in relation to goods such as skin care products which are purchased not just for beautification but more usually with the intention of self-medication.

The ACA criticized the way the industry cons the public into believing that various products have been independently assessed and found useful and, after dissecting the texts of various adverts for skin care products, said:

> Such claims are misleading as they imply that there is a professionally agreed opinion as to therapeutic effect when in fact authorative professional bodies, such as the Australasia College of Dermatologists may dispute the claims or hold no settled opinion as to the benefits claimed. Foods, medicines, and dental products making health claims may not obtain a false authority by references to members of health professions or institutions and this has assisted in protecting consumers from exposure to charlatan claims. On the other hand, cosmetics manufacturers have licence to imply academic validity which may be misleading. Many consumers may misconstrue references to scientific tests as being independently conducted when in fact they are conducted by company employees or client organizations.

The ACA ended up making no fewer than 25 different recommendations of ways in which the industry could be made to sharpen up its act and which would give the customer greater protection from false or misleading claims.

In this country, cosmetics, unlike food, do not have to be labelled and, because they can contain up to 10,000 different ingredients, we have no way of assessing the effectiveness (or true cost) of what is in the bottle.

If you *do* find out what's in the products, some of the ingredients make unpleasant reading. In chapter six I will look at the use of animals both as a source of ingredients and for safety testing. Many buyers of cosmetics may find some of these practices an unacceptable price to pay for their hygiene and, let's face it, their vanity.

THE ANTI-AGEING BONANZA

From time to time, the cosmetics industry surpasses itself. A recent example of this has been the anti-ageing bonanza. For women mostly, although not exclusively, this has meant expensive skin-creams, and for men (again mostly, but not exclusively), this has meant new tonics designed to restore thinning hair. The latter have fallen into the realms of drugs, and therefore, unlike cosmetics and most other hair preparations, are open to independent scientific evaluation. Chapter fifteen looks at the rapidly expanding market of cosmetics for men.

However much we stay out of the sun, however much we cut down on alcohol, smoking, coffee, late nights and improve our intake of food, fresh air and clean living, however much we apply expensive creams, we cannot halt the ravages of time. The years of living life to the full etch lines too deep to be removed by anything other than a scalpel. Chapter eighteen looks at the world of cosmetic surgery which reaches the parts that anti-ageing creams claim to (but cannot possibly) reach, to see how it works and whether it is worth it.

Thankfully, some fads fall by the wayside. A vogue in the early 1980s was for 'laser treatments' — the surgical removal of crow's feet by small lasers. This treatment was available in many high street salons. Highly risky, especially to the eyeball itself, as well as the delicate skin around the eyes, these potential weapons were being wielded by many unskilled beauticians as if they were make-up pencils.

No doubt there are a few places where you can still get this kind of treatment, but a generally bad press by Fleet Street — but not by the beauty editors of course — and warnings from ophthalmologists have saved many from potential danger (and not inconsiderable expense).

From time to time, stories crop up, again in the newspapers (which aren't dependent on cosmetic advertising), about the dangers of certain types of cosmetics, or beauty practices. A recent one was the revelation by the *Daily Mirror* that electrolysis was being practised by 'technicians' who had undergone a mere four weeks all-round beauty training, and a number of clients had been scarred for life as a result.

On the whole, beauty salons, health farms and hairdressers have too much to lose by employing unskilled staff and offering sharp practices. But if you have had a bad experience you should always complain, and not merely to the salon itself, but to some regulatory authority like the Department of Trade or your local council Trading Standards officer to try to ensure that other people do not suffer in the same way.

If you have a bad experience with a hairdresser or beauty practitioner, complain to your local Council Trading Standards Officer. Don't let others suffer, too!

As for the products themselves, again, cosmetics and toiletries rarely kill, unless seriously misused. But, as a lawyer acting for Ralph Nader's Public Citizen, an active consumer group in America recently said:

There almost never will be a documented case where someone died because of Red No 3 (a colour additive) in lipstick. People are exposed to so many carcinogens that you can't say which one caused cancer. But just because there are no identifiable victims doesn't mean that it's safe.

Last year, the consumer group challenged the cosmetics industry in the American courts over the continued presence of two dyes used very widely indeed in the industry, Red No 19 and Orange No 17. Both were known to have caused liver cancer in rats in experiments carried out by the cosmetics industry.

The industry responded by arguing that it was ten times safer to use a lipstick containing Red No 19 for a *lifetime* than to *occasionally* eat a charcoal-broiled steak. Since many women do use a favourite lipstick for a lifetime, and possibly other cosmetics containing carcinogenic dyes as well, this defensive argument lacks force.

NO WARNINGS FROM THE INDUSTRY

As I will elaborate in the chapter on hair dyes, two Irish women have recently died as a result of cancer caused by repeatedly dyeing their hair, in a case widely unreported, yet highly significant for the industry and for any woman who regularly dyes her hair at home, or has it done in a salon.

> 'Just because there are no identifiable victims doesn't mean that it's safe'.
> *Public Citizen lawyer*

Does the industry warn us about these things? No, it keeps quiet. Occasionally it changes the products — for example by bringing pale lipsticks or different hair colours into fashion, but we have to discover any hazards for ourselves, and then usually only by trial and error. That means wasting our money and breaking out in rashes and spots.

Americans seem obsessed with consumerism and suing one another. In Britain, we are almost the opposite. We are a willing, docile breed content to be duped by the ad-men, conned by the industry and frightened to stand up for ourselves and ask any of the right questions.

This book will, I hope, tackle some of these questions and offer at least some of the answers. No-one teaches us about cosmetics before we set off at an early age to start buying and using them and a greedy and competitive industry preys on our insecurity and ignorance.

CHAPTER ONE

THE HISTORY: NOTHING IS REALLY 'NEW' IN COSMETICS

Although fashions change, women throughout the centuries have always wanted the same things: soft, smooth, youthful skins, rosy lips and cheeks, large seductive eyes and soft, feminine, flattering hair. Men, on the other hand, have always wanted to look strong, and capable of being breadwinners, whether they were primitive hunters caked in woad, medieval courtiers with prospects of political influence and wealth, or latter-day chaps worth knowing and eventually marrying.

We have historical evidence that the use of make up and cosmetics goes back at least 5,000 years. Archaeologists have found, for example, remains of lip rouge from that far back. From surviving Greek statues, we know that popular images of beauty have remained remarkably unchanged. Teenage magazines and Mills and Boon novels still depict the desirable male or female face in classical proportions, with a straight aquiline nose, wide forehead and large eyes and lips.

ROMANS AND BEAUTY

Because we have a lot of evidence of what happened in Roman times, we known that Roman men and women were as preoccupied with their looks as we are today, and that they employed a host of strategems to enhance their natural beauty. In fact, a typical fashionable Roman lady would not look seriously out of place if she walked down a modern High Street, except perhaps for her clothes.

Roman women lavishly applied perfumes to their bodies, not because they wanted, as their descendants did during later decades, to disguise their body odours, but because they were scrupulous about bathing and hygiene. However, we might well wonder how

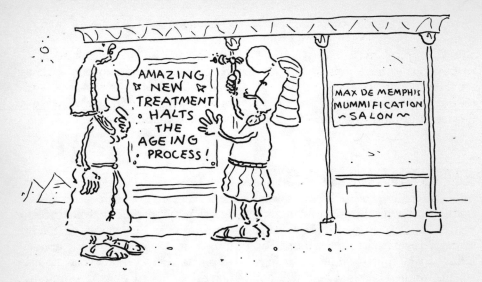

effective their night-creams were, as they were made from a rather revolting gluey paste of flour and milk.

They used depilatories, hair dyes, skin creams and acne potions, along with tooth whiteners and toothpastes made from a concoction of horn, pumice stone or a mixture of potassium and sodium carbonate (salt).

The eye make-up they used then is still copied today, in the form of kohl which can be used inside the rims of the eyes. They also used burnt cork as a kind of mascara on their eyelashes.

They had eyebrow tweezers which were not only used by the ladies to pluck their eyebrows, but also by men to trim their facial hair. Indeed, it is said that Julius Caesar used to have his barb-er or 'tonsor' pluck all his facial hairs out individually! The Emperor Nero apparently used cosmetics like kohl for his eyes, ceruse (white lead) and chalk to whiten his skin, rouge on his lips and cheeks and a pumice stone to whiten his teeth.

We know that Cleopatra bathed in asses' milk, and her maids spent hours braiding her hair and making her skin silken and beautiful and her eyes dark and sultry enough to win Anthony. She used all sorts of colours to emphasize her eyes and lips and whitened her face with chalk.

In ancient Egypt, crocodile dung was found to be an excellent face-mask. Presumably it is only a matter of time before a modern cosmetic house rediscovers the formula, corners the supply of this ingredient from the banks of the world's tropical rivers and we are all rushing out to the shops to buy it!

Little make-up was used in Europe after the fall of the Roman Empire in the fifth century until the Crusaders start-ed bringing back cosmetics and perfumes from the East. They were more popular on the continent and at the French court than in England until the reign of Elizabeth I. Until then, cosmetics were used only by harlots to cover their pock-marked faces.

THE MIDDLE AGES

In the Middle Ages, in most parts of the world, women strove to look pale and wan and the portraits of the time show fashionable women with no hint of personality in their elongated oval faces. It is hard to guess whether this was the fashionable look to adopt or simply the accepted style for portrait painters.

They looked rather severe because of the practice of not only plucking out all of the eyebrows, but also the hairs on their temples and necks, to emphasize their elaborate headdresses. Women with beautiful eyes got away with this look, but plainer types ended up looking rather vacant and stupid. The hair was rarely flattering, but pulled back sharply from the face, so the colour was a harsh outline rather than a soft frame.

Women used many devices to make themselves look pale: they swallowed gravel, ashes, candle wax, or even arsenic, most of which, not surprisingly, made them look very weak and sickly indeed. Some women even tried washing in their own urine to drain their colour and yet others used strips of bacon on their faces at night! Because all this made the skin's condition rather poor, medication was used in the form of asparagus roots, asses' and goats' milk and the bulbs of white lilies, aged in horse manure.

ELIZABETHAN TIMES

Elizabeth, who was 25 when she came to the throne in 1558, was both vain and insecure. She made most of her own cosmetics. Ingredients included pigeons' wings and claws, beetle blood, turpentine, eggs, honey, shells, ground mother-of-pearl, musk (from deer) and amber-gris (from whales). Until her reign only perfumes and pommanders were in widespread use in fashionable society, mainly to ward off body odours. Perfumed gloves were also fashionable.

In general, hygiene was not considered important and, depending on which history books you read, Queen Elizabeth is said at best to have bathed only once a month, and at worst, to have only taken one bath in her entire life.

DEADLY PALE

The Queen made fashionable the widespread use of ceruse (white lead), which was made into face powder and rouge. It was mixed with egg-white and gave the wearer a mask-like appearance.

This practice was literally deadly, and women who used ceruse rarely kept their looks past the age of thirty. The fashionable ghostly white complexion of the Middle Ages was even more damaging to the skin than the fashionable tan of the twentieth century. Excessive use of white lead could kill, and many aristocratic beauties of the later Middle Ages, whose portraits remain, went to an early grave in the name of vanity. One of the most famous of these was the Countess of Coventry who perished at the age of 27 because she stubbornly insisted on covering her beautiful face with ceruse and using mercuric substances on her skin and lips.

Following the fashion at court was everything to these ladies. For example, when Elizabeth began to lose her hair, she started to wear wigs, and ladies of fashion copied her example, along with painting veins on their brows to show 'breeding' and class.

Poisonous substances were commonplace in the cosmetics then available. For example, in his book of *Fashions in Make Up: From Ancient to Modern Times* (Owen 1972), Richard Corson tells how, in Italy, in the seventeenth century, a 'cosmetic preparation' was sold with verbal instructions very different from those written on the bottle and it was not until more than six hundred husbands had died of arsenic poisoning that Mrs Toffana was arrested and executed as the most wicked mass murderess of her time.

PATCHES FOR POCK MARKS

In the seventeenth century the wearing of facial patches became popular to hide the pock-marks which most people possessed. Patches were made from black or red leather or silk in various shapes and were stuck to the skin with gum. Samuel Pepys and his wife wore patches and his diaries describe his admiration for the fashion.

When rich men and women lost their teeth, they wore 'plumpers', small discs of cork or leather, in their mouths, to keep their cheeks looking fashionably full. Because toothpastes of the time contained sulphuric and nitric acids, they destroyed the enamel and hence few people in fashionable society had a full set of teeth. False teeth made of wood or bone were wired into place. Men and women who wore plumpers and false teeth tended to talk with a lisp and so lisping became a sign of good breeding.

False eyebrows were often worn because the ceruse make-up eventually destroyed the natural ones. These were made from mouse skin and often worn quite high on the forehead, which explains why portraits of many fashionable people of the time show them with a rather surprised look.

Because the lives of the rich and the poor were so very different, their appearance was very dissimilar. Only the rich had access to wigs and patches and face make-up to disguise their scars, blemishes and natural defects.

The poor, by contrast, and as depicted in Hogarth's paintings, suffered from malnutrition, poor health, and were worn to a frazzle by constant (and frequently unsuccessful) pregnancies, and by incessant gin-drinking. Only peasants and gypsies had healthy suntanned complexions of the kind we admire today.

By the end of the seventeenth century, men and women openly wore make-up, especially at court. Judge Jeffreys, Lord Chancellor of England, was said to have worn make-up quite flagrantly.

As an indication of how much rouge was worn, it was estimated in 1781 that French women used two million pots of rouge a year with a range of more than a dozen different varieties.

Other cosmetics tricks of the time included darkening the eyebrows with crushed elderberries or charcoal, and dyeing the hair with walnut leaves and black lead. Recipes for skin creams included ingredients such as 'macerated sheep's marrow, sheep's trotters and calves feet, together with sheep's wax (lanolin), kid's grease and borax'. Before you start feeling too squeamish, remember that many of today's most expensive skin creams contain similar, albeit more attractive-sounding ingredients.

The use of cosmetics and artificial devices was so common and so controversial that, at the end of the eighteenth century, Parliament passed an act which made it illegal to 'seduce into matrimony by the use of scents, paints, cosmetics, artificial teeth, false hair . . . or bolstered hips'. Men it seems, were tired of being tricked by false visions of what they were actually attaching themselves to! Although the law was pretty unenforceable, gradually the excessive use of make-up went out of fashion.

There were frequent criticisms of the over-use of rouge, and the combined effect of bright red blobs on chalk-white cheeks, together with no emphasis on the eyes appears to us now — and many people then — as far too clownish, and very unappealing. However, since after dark this garish make-up was only seen under the softening effects of candle-light, perhaps it did not seem so bad.

THE VICTORIAN VIEW

Later on, in the Victorian era, middle-class women did not openly wear make-up — once again it was mostly for the trollops.

Ladies pinched their cheeks to create a 'blush' — rouge was completely out of fashion — and young ladies did exercises to try to alter their mouths into the fashionable puckered shape. Pale faces were still fashionable and some occasionally resorted to using a palatte of rice powder. Cosmetic products sold for 'health' purposes, like lip salves, were acceptable, and some had an added hint of colour, but one of the most shameful things a society female could admit to was wearing make up. Victorian beauty experts were wise enough to warn about the dangers of using lead-based make-up and hair dyes.

A substitute was found at last for the lethal white lead in the form of bismuth-oxychloride which, although non-poisonous, had the unfortunate side-effect of turning black when worn in a smokey room! Thus, on cold winter nights in front of warm blazing fires, many a fashionably pale lady of the time turned an embarrassing greyish-black during the course of the evening!

Make-up was frowned on but hair, by contrast, was elaborate and pretty and was curled in to ringlets to frame the face; hairpieces were commonly used.

BEAUTY AND BLACKMAIL

Perhaps the most famous entrepreneur in the emerging cosmetics business of Victorian times was Madame Rachel, who opened a beauty parlour in Bond Street in 1863. She charged an astonishing fee of one thousand guineas or more for her course of beauty baths, but her avarice led her into blackmailing her customers by threatening to tell their husbands (and prim Victorian society in general) what they were up to. She was tried and convicted for fraud and sentenced to five years in prison and her fantastically successful business collapsed. Amongst other things, she sold 'Jordan Water' which was guaranteed to keep the skin young, even though it came from a pump in the back yard.

Another 'rip-off' of the times was exposed in a legal fight over the patent for a popular lotion which sold for seven shillings and sixpence a pint. Investigation revealed that the ingredients, mainly water and bitter almonds, cost two pence and the bottle three pence — a mark-up of 1,700 per cent!

An article in *The Cornhill Magazine* in the 1860s stated candidly 'fortunes are made by cosmetics', whilst another article in the *Athenaeum* condemned those mothers who applied white make-up to their children's faces. Intelligent opinion was that crude application of unnatural face powders was foolish and unattractive.

Affluent Victorians truly believed that 'cleanliness was next to Godliness' and daily bathing became routine in households that could afford the soap and servants to bring up the water jugs. In 1876, only half of London's houses had a constant water supply and most people lived in such terrible conditions that beauty was the last thing they worried about.

BEGINNINGS OF THE COSMETIC INDUSTRY

Things began to change towards the end of the nineteenth century as the restrictiveness of the Victorian era eased up. The foundations of the modern cosmetics industry were laid and companies like those started by Jesse Boot began to make cosmetics the poor could afford, through mass production techniques. It was about this time that soap began to be manufactured commercially. By 1900, there were over 120 branches of Boots. Cyclax, one of the first companies to concentrate on making cosmetics, started up in 1886. The rise of the big beauty houses began in America, Paris and London. The founders are not forgotten for their names still appear on many products sold today.

In America, beauty salons began to flourish from the 1880s onwards but they did not catch on in Britain until much later. The census of 1849 records that there were already 39 cosmetic companies in America. This did not include the 'quacks' who went round the country on horseback selling their dubious pills and potions. At this time the country's total outlay on cosmetics was still very modest but by 1915, Americans were buying £50 million dollars' worth of cosmetics a year.

Yardley was exporting more than twenty different kinds of soap to America, and won awards for its 'Brown Windsor' brand at the Great Exhibition of 1851 — an event which stimulated the cosmetics and toiletries industry. Yardley set up their London perfume factory in Bloomsbury in 1883. The top English companies competed for space in fashionable Bond Street.

In Paris, Monsieur Coty tried to persuade a store to sell his home-made perfume and was refused. As he left, he managed to smash the bottle and the smell that escaped was so delicious to the curious customers who surrounded him that he was immediately given his first order.

In 1899, Harriet Hubbard Ayer made a successful start in the beauty business by launching a white foundation liquid to replace enamelling substances. She took on a partner called Florence Nightingale Graham, but the working partnership lasted only a short while. Changing her name to Elizabeth Arden, Mrs Graham set up on her own with a borrowed $6,000. The rest is history — Elizabeth Arden herself is no longer alive, but her world-famous company prospers, albeit now owned and run by men in the pharmaceutical industry.

Interestingly, the Edwardian times were the only period of history in which women tried to look middle-aged, because it was realized that older women appealed to the Prince of Wales, who was a tremendous trendsetter.

BETWEEN THE WARS

The main cosmetic development of the First World War was the emergence of plastic surgeons who began face and body reconstruction to repair the horrific war-wounds men (and a few women) had sustained. This laid the foundations of the cosmetic surgery industry that does so well in affluent parts of the world today.

After the First World War, women not only felt more liberated, but also found that eligible men were in very short supply. In this very different era, make up became acceptable to all classes and the spreading of mass-market chain stores like Woolworths made cosmetics cheap and readily available.

In higher social circles, young 'flappers' flaunted their made-up looks and tweezered their eyebrows into delicate arches familiar to us through the *Vogue* magazine pictures of the era. The first 'twist-up' lipstick was patented in 1915, and these, along with smoking and cigarette-holders, became the accessories of the 'flappers'. Cosmetics companies were even making waterproof rouge.

According to magazines like *Vogue*, it was as essential for women to wear make-up during the 1920s as it had been *not* to do so only a generation before.

When Max Factor started business in 1936, many office girls spent most of their weekly wages on clothes and cosmetics, copying the looks of Hollywood idols like Jean Harlow, Greta Garbo and Marlene Deitrich. The screen idols became the symbols of beauty to replace the actresses and aristocratic beauties of former centuries.

For the first time, magazines showed ordinary girls and women how they could look like film-stars. While Arden and Rubenstein began their legendary battle for the number one position in the skincare industry, new firms like Almay, Clairol, Goya, Germaine Monteuil and Wella were starting up.

THE FASHION FOR TANS

Because everyone could now afford to buy cosmetics, the wealthy had to find something else to set them apart from the common tribe. It was at this time that suntans were made fashionable by Coco Chanel, and because only the rich could afford to travel to the sun to acquire the necessary glow. Salons specialized in removing a sallowing suntan with bleach treatments.

Sales of cosmetics had taken off so dramatically that it was estimated that every woman in America was spending £15 a head per year, and that did not include soaps or perfumes. Ten years later, the sales figures had quadrupled. It was reckoned that the average American woman spent £50 dollars per year on cosmetics and treatments, which was more than the average man was spending on tobacco. By the time of the Wall Street Crash in 1929, one advertising agency calculated that American women were using the equivalent of three thousand miles of lipstick a year — enough, end to end, to bridge London and New York!

THE SECOND WORLD WAR AND AFTER

During the Second World War, cosmetics were naturally in short supply. Factories were producing war supplies — not trivial things like make up. Factory girls dreamed about looking beautiful again and many women fell back on home-made remedies or the black market, and delved deep into their dressing table stocks.

After the Second World War the cosmetics industry really took off. Women not only had jobs and were earning good money which they wanted to spend on new things, but also they were anxious to employ all the beauty tricks the magazines could offer them to look attractive for their husbands and lovers when they returned from the front. The fashion was for women to have large breasts and a shapely hour glass figure. Make up was cheap and readily available, and was used fairly unsubtly, with bright red lipstick all the rage.

By the 1950s, the eyes had become more important than the lips, and subtler shades of lipstick were used. Eyeliner came in and was applied enthusiastically.

In the 1960s and 1970s, the feminist movement began, and its most ardent supporters symbolically threw away their feminine adornments, including make up, and wore their hair long and loose with straggly ends, or cropped short, like men's.

It was fashionable to have large black-rimmed eyes, framed by long, straight honey blonde hair and women whose hair was unfashionably curly spent hours ironing and straightening out their curls whilst many others peroxided their hair to look as much as they could like the most popular female figures of the time — Brigitte Bardot, Jean Shrimpton, Twiggy and Julie Christie.

Messy, unkempt hairstyles hinted at a liberated lifestyle complete with late nights, drink, drugs and rock and roll — even if the reality was that most of these models and actresses were routinely having early nights to keep up with the rigours of their occupation. False eyelashes were commonly worn, both above and below the eye, and teenagers began to spend hours on their faces before going out.

There was even a craze for freckles and those with none of their own were encouraged to dot some artificial ones on their cheeks to achieve the desired effect.

THE SEVENTIES AND EIGHTIES

The 1970s and 1980s have been characterized by a return to more natural looks, and the most admired women are those, like Jane Fonda, who exemplify fitness and healthiness rather than the use of heavy make up. Indeed, many models have appeared on magazine covers wearing little or no make up, to the consternation of the cosmetics companies.

When *Elle* was launched in Britain in the mid 1980s, it regularly featured models wearing little or no make up, and in beauty features its emphasis was on looking healthy rather than looking cosmetically 'perfect'. Fashion photographer David Bailey refers to this breed of models as the clean-faced 'vegetarian' girls, a far cry from the traditionally beautiful women who escort him.

Manufacturers have responded to this trend by making a vast range of 'natural', 'organic', 'herbal' and 'biological' products designed to appeal to the cosmetic-buying women of today. Synthetic artificial products are 'out' and anything natural is 'in'. There is no 'look' which is *the* look. Girls wearing no make-up mix with punks wearing warpaint and hairstyles streaked in primary colours. Singers like Boy George emphasize the fact that men are once again beginning to wear cosmetics and fiddle around with their hair.

In the world of beauty, and the cosmetics which enhance it, it seems that nothing is new despite incessant minor changes by the trend-setters in the business. The concepts themselves are as old as human vanity.

CHAPTER TWO

THE PSYCHOLOGY OF BEAUTY AND THE COSMETICS INDUSTRY

It is tempting to dismiss the use of cosmetics as utterly trivial, but research shows that an individual's physical appearance has a substantial effect on his or her life.

Studies show that attractive people enjoy many advantages, including greater self-confidence and self-esteem, popularity with friends, ease of getting on in the jobs and activities they choose and an ability to marry higher in the social scale than their less attractive associates. What's more, people attribute additional qualities to attractive people which they do not bestow on plainer individuals.

FIRST IMPRESSIONS ARE VITAL

Alarmingly perhaps, we assess each other's attractiveness during the first four minutes of the initial meeting, according to studies carried out by American psychologist, Leonard Zunin.

Although the finding is true of men too, it is women who spend vast amounts of time and money on cosmetics and treatments designed to improve on nature, whilst men, generally speaking, are urged to prove themselves in other ways, either academically or athletically at school, and afterwards by affluence — smart cars, for example.

Even so, regardless of how much they achieve in other ways, attractive men, like beautiful women, are always given a headstart in life.

Interestingly, when asked what attracts them towards men when they first meet, 30 per cent of women notice the eyes, whilst only 22 per cent of men notice women's eyes. And whilst 27 per cent of women are first attracted by a man's face, 34 per cent of men notice this first about the women they meet. Women are more aware of men's smiles and teeth than vice-versa and men pay more attention to women's figures and legs than women do of men's. However, the sexes apparently pay equal attention to each other's hairstyle, along with hair colour.

Most people agree that the skilful use of cosmetics can improve the looks of that vast majority of us who are not born naturally beautiful. Make-up *does* enable women to camouflage their bad features and enhance the good ones, increasing their chances of approval from teachers, employers, social contacts, and above all, the opposite sex.

HIDING BEHIND MAKE-UP

Many women go so far in their use of make-up that each day they put on a daily 'mask' for the world. Some women spend 20 minutes in the bathroom each morning 'putting on their face' and they find it inconceivable that other women will appear wearing no make-up at all.

I feel rather sorry for the women who even dress and make up for bed, or who are careful to put the light out before facing their loved one stripped of all make-up. It must occur to them that sometime he is bound to get a glimpse of the real them, complete with blotchy skin and bags and wrinkles, and the more they cake on the make-up, the

greater the shock when the truth is revealed.

Everything these women do to arrange their looks is a projection of the way they want the world to see them — from the carefully highlighted and shaped style of their hair to the ends of their manicured fingertips. The image does not necessarily reflect what they are like inside, but it is what they want to display to others and indicates how they want to be treated.

Wearing no make-up, unless you are very young, can draw as negative a reaction from people around you as wearing too much make-up. There is a delicate balance to be achieved somehow between these extremes. In this way, we can wear make-up and toiletries to give us the confidence of feeling fresh and at our best, without feeling we are hiding behind an image of someone else we create each time we look in the mirror, with brushes and pots and tubes in hand.

For most of us, it is acceptable to look as though we care about our appearance and have made some effort to look nice. However, this should be achieved without having to whisk out a lipstick or powder compact every five minutes. Anyone who finds it inconceivable to face the world without ritually (re-)applying a public mask, almost certainly has a deeper problem which is well beyond the scope of this book.

An interesting study of attitudes

towards cosmetics was carried out in Britain by an American cosmetics company in 1978. It revealed that many women felt they did not *exist* when they did not wear make-up. When asked for a one-word description of how they felt, bereft of cosmetics, the women replied 'frumpy', 'terrible', 'dowdy' and 'ghastly'.

MAKE-UP AND LIFESTYLE

A lot depends, of course, on a woman's lifestyle, and in particular whether she goes out to work or not. Women who go out to work each day often feel they owe it to their bosses, colleagues, and most importantly, to themselves, to look smart. Women who work in factories are less likely to be bothered about their work image than women working as receptionists, personal secretaries, waitresses, stewardesses or shop assistants. But the factory worker may care very much what her male and female colleagues think of her appearance.

On the other hand, women who do not go out to work but who stay at home bringing up children much more reliant on make-up and their image because they are no independent status other than as wives and mothers.

Jean Graham, a social psychologist in Professor Kligman's Department of Dermatology at the University of Pennsylvania, has specialized in studying the psychology of women and cosmetics, and she has consistently found that when women wear make-up they are more confident, efficient and outgoing than when they wear nothing on their faces. Not surprisingly, her research has made her very popular with the cosmetics industry and she is in great demand to lecture all over America on the psychological merits of using cosmetics.

PSYCHOTHERAPEUTIC COSMETOLOGY

Jean Graham has also found that cosmetics can be very therapeutic psychologically, and has done research with groups of women in their sixties who were either ill in hospital or suffering from emotional disorders. She found that teaching women — especially those who had never used such things before — to apply skin creams and make-up not only improved their self-esteem but also their whole outlook and sense of optimism. The results were particularly significant amongst those women who had never considered themselves attractive, for whom the 'makeovers' provided a new lease of life. Many could not wait to leave their sick beds to show their 'new' faces to the world.

Other research by the Red Cross has shown that the use of cosmetics and hairdressing skills can help speed the recovery of sick and bedridden patients by promoting feelings of psychological well-being.

'Psychotherapeutic cosmetology', as it is called, is relatively new, but the signs are that cosmetics and beauty therapies such as massage could have an increasing role to play in future health care. Many companies are already cashing in on the vogue for 'aromatherapy', in which oils and scents are used to increase feelings of well-being.

Professor Albert Kligman of the University of Pennsylvania, believes that good looks have assumed greater importance because this is the television age, and we have become much more visually orientated.

In his book, *The Psychology of Cosmetic Treatments* (Praegar), he says:

Physicians have long appreciated society's cruel aversive behaviour to those with deformities. There is a huge [amount of] literature dealing with the plight of the physically handicapped, the crippled, the hunchback, the congenitally deformed and the like. Yet doctors have not been fully enlightened on the predicament of 'normal' people who happen to be physically unattractive . . . Study after study has demonstrated that that the physically unattractive are disadvantaged, in education, in jobs, in romance, in marriage, even in such places as the mental hospital and the courtroom.

Beauty may be skin deep but ugliness is bone deep, a serious handicap in pursuit of health and happiness. Indeed, there is some evidence that the physically unattractive enjoy poorer physical health and well-being.

In Professor Kligman's view it is a myth that beauty is in the eye of the beholder and this is perhaps so, for whereas we vary from one another in our assessment of the attractiveness of others, for the most part we can all broadly agree on who we consider to be truly beautiful.

Professor Kligman has devoted his career to dermatology and how to understand and improve the quality of the skin. And it is the skin, the body's largest organ, and its covering of the face in particular, which is the foundation of beauty.

Perhaps this is not so surprising when you consider that it is through face to face contact that the vast majority of human relationships are initiated, and it is the features we focus on as we get to know one another.

It seems grossly unfair that beautiful people can often get away with being quite dismissive and unpleasant to others, whilst ugly people can be the nicest individuals you'll ever meet and yet be discounted as friends, socially ostracized and overlooked in their work — particularly if they are women.

To prove that our concept of what constitutes beauty is universal, research by Michael Cunningham at the University of Louisville in Kentucky found highly consistent results.

When a group of 150 white male undergraduates were asked to rate the attractiveness of 50 women from pictures of their faces, certain common findings emerged. He found that the eyes had to be three-tenths of the width of the face, the chin length one fifth the length of the face overall, and the total area of the nose less than five per cent of the face.

When analysed in this way, it was found that if, for example a woman's mouth was less than 50 per cent of the width of the face at mouth level, then she was generally perceived as being less attractive than other women with more generous mouths, but that women with very large mouths were also deemed less attractive.

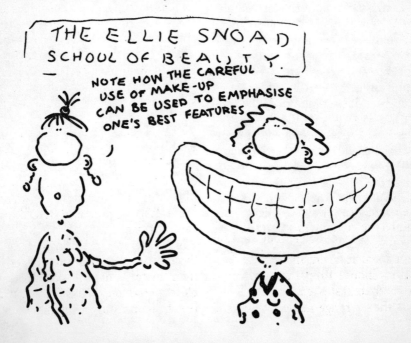

GET THEM YOUNG

The cosmetics industry knows that 20 per cent of the female population is aged between 15 and 20 and also that girls start wearing make-up regularly from the age of 13 or younger (and that most women don't stop until they are too old to see what they are doing — if then!).

The teen market is profitable and the youngsters worth exploiting (or catering for, depending on which way you look at it). In Britain, teenagers spend about £25 million a year on cosmetics, of which about a quarter goes on fragrances alone.

Despite the recession, and youth unemployment, this age group spends a very great deal of its spare cash on cosmetics and clothes. Perhaps if you can't get a job and you don't have heavy financial responsibilities, satisfaction can be derived from looking good and (therefore?) feeling great. This way of thinking is rigorously endorsed by the teenage magazines, which emphasize not how to accept yourself as you are, but how to improve upon what you were born with.

The cosmetics industry believes that if it grabs the customers when they are still young and impressionable, they'll remain loyal forever, and can always pick and choose from the company's range as their tastes change.

Thus the *17* range made by Boots is very important to the company and is constantly bringing out new colours and exciting and desirable products designed to appeal to the girl with pocket or Saturday-job money at her disposal. The *Miners* collection is produced by Max Factor — another company which directs a great deal of their products at teenagers. They are aware that in order to keep the customers interested they have to continually bring out new colours, because experimentation is what teenage make up is all about. For this reason, assistants working on counters displaying teenage cosmetics are instructed not to interfere unless specifically asked for advice or information. 'Children' need their playground, and deliberating over the choice of a product and soliciting companions' approval is part of the fun and is crucial in making a sale.

Older customers either know exactly what they want, or are less conscious about the impression the very latest colour is going to make on their circle of friends or colleagues — who, unlike the teenagers, probably don't know or care anyway.

Adolescents are horrified by the thought of seeming out of step with their mates, and the cosmetics (and clothes) industry plays on this insecurity by constantly bringing out 'new' products, a good example being the frosted white mascara which was a recent rage. Adolesence is an extraordinary time, both of rebellion against authority and of extreme conformity to 'the look' deemed to be 'in' at the time. Both boys and girls become very narcissistic at this age.

The fact that there are only a handful of girls in every generation who have the kind of beauty that sets all pulses racing and stops traffic in the streets does not prevent moderately attractive young girls hoping that, if they can only find the right blusher, the right eyeshadow and achieve the perfect delicately suntanned skin, they, too, may become a stunning beauty.

TINY TOTS AND BABIES

The industry also caters for the very young — babies have their own ranges of toiletries, geared towards nappy rash and cleanliness rather than beauty, and there are still 'beautiful baby' contests at many village fêtes, designed to appeal to mothers' fantasies of having given birth to a future beauty queen. On a national scale, there is the 'Miss Pears' annual contest, and recently companies like Peaudouce, who make nappies, have started to run tiny tots contests using the most appealing little boys and girls they can find. So far, the British have not gone as far as the Americans. One American mother dressed her two-year-old up in false eyelashes before entering her in a 'beauty contest'.

From about five upwards, little girls often start imitating their mothers, wanting to wear lipsticks and perfumes. Not surprisingly, there are make-up ranges designed specifically for the very young, usually at disproportionately high prices — a lipstick in a tiny tot make-up kit commonly costs more than the average adult brand. Make-up specifically for children is preferable to adult make-up, if kids insist they want to wear it, for example, 'nail varnish' which can be peeled off instead of needing potentially lethal acetone nail varnish remover to remove it.

Children's toys also pander to the image of female beauty, with Barbie Dolls and the like which have ridiculous hour glass shapes and perfect blonde flicked-up hair, rosebud mouths and true blue eyes. Little girls can have make-up and hairdressing sets for their dolls to accustom them to the habit, in later years, of manicuring themselves along the same lines.

By the time these children get to school, they are already aware of the importance of looking attractive. Psychologists have found that even from the age of five children start to discriminate between ugly and attractive people. Pretty girls have more friends than plain ones and get more fuss at school from teachers and at home from parents and relatives.

SELF-ESTEEM

Women's sometimes obsessive preoccupation with how they look was explored by Nancy Baker in her book *The Beauty Trap* (Piatkus, 1986). She described how, when she was about to appear on national television in America, the thing which worried both herself and her friends was not what she would *say*, but how she would *look*.

Although she was on television to promote a serious book she had just written exposing scandals in black market adoption, she was astonished at how she and her friends had all trivialized the occasion. Friends advised her on what to wear, how to do her make-up and what to do with her hair. Afterwards their comments were all purely about her *appearance* — what she had said seemingly provoked no reaction from them. After the publicity tour was over,
she realized she too had fallen into what she called the 'beauty trap'. She said, 'I let my appearance assume far too much importance in my life. I attached unrealistic expectations to beauty. And, when I looked in the mirror, I didn't like what I saw.'

If you think about it, it is strange that despite women's lib and all that has followed, we still do not appear to have moved far from Jane Austen's day, especially when you observe how a pretty sister/daughter/friend is still treated by her acquaintances. She may be bright, or even brilliant, and/or she may be athletic, but others (men and women) will still speculate on her behalf — often quite openly — about the rich, handsome and very eligible man she will no doubt win in the marriage and social stakes.

NO WOMAN IS HAPPY WITH HER LOOKS

One rather extraordinary fact, revealed in various pieces of research, is that nearly *all* women are dissatisfied with their looks, regardless of their class or level of intelligence, and they worry to a greater or lesser extent about trying to improve them.

A study published in the *Journal of the American Dietetic Association* in 1980
noted that 91 per cent of high-achieving female students interviewed by researchers at New York University were dissatisfied with their bodies and their looks. Actresses, film stars and models all have doubts about their appearance and would like to change various features of it. It is perhaps comforting to know that it is not just ordinary

women who worry about their looks, but many of the world's most beautiful women, too.

Men worry about these things but to a much lesser extent. (After all, as one — rather unattractive — middle-aged man once bragged to me, 'Men mature, women age.') Men worry about losing their hair, mainly because they think that is associated with a loss of virility, not because they dread no longer looking young. They rarely worry about wrinkles, unless they are ageing executives still hoping for promotion (See chapter eighteen on cosmetic surgery).

Research shows that, earlier on in life, ugliness is an important factor, and one theory is that juvenile delinquents often act that way because they are ugly. Society rejects them and cuts them off if they are physically unattractive and their work is, often unfairly, judged to be inferior. Ugly people, male and female, are often thought of poorly, and their genuine good qualities are overlooked. This can set up a vicious circle as they may feel bitter, and believe that since nobody loves them anyway they may as well start becoming unlovable.

RESEARCH PROVES THE POINT

These theories about attractiveness were tested in a study in New York in which a group of male undergraduates were given an essay to 'mark'. Two essays were used in the test, one was poorly written and the other rather well written. Attached to both essays were photos of the alleged authors, one attractive and the other rather plain.

Although the good essay generally received better marks, there was a significant tendency for those students who had been given the poor essay to still give a high mark providing the photo of the pretty girl was attached. Similarly, the well-written essay

was commended less when it was attached to the photo of the unattractive author.

The researchers then carried out a similar experiment to see how physical appearance affects people's chances of getting a job. They gave fake job applications to 80 different employers, together with pictures of the supposed applicants. The attractive applicants were rated more positively and were definitely given greater chances of an interview, despite the fact that their qualifications were no better than the less attractive applicants who were given the thumbs-down.

BUT WHY IS PHYSICAL BEAUTY SO IMPORTANT?

Darwin put his finger on it of course — the purpose of beauty in the animal world is to attract a mate and thus ensure survival of the species. Unfortunately for women, it is traditional in the human race for females to dress up and appeal to the males, unlike in many of the lower species, such as birds, where it is the other way round. Just look at the boring old peahen alongside the magnificent peacock, or the dull old brown female pheasant, alongside her dazzling gold and emerald male suitors. Or even — despite her beautiful dark brown eyes — the timid roe deer, alongside the magnificent antlered buck. However, there are signs of a change among humans: men are becoming increasingly vain.

Throughout the centuries, for the vast majority of women, survival and the material quality of life has depended almost wholly on attracting a male and finding a partner for life with whom to breed. The more beautiful the woman, the richer the pickings. We can all see that Prince Charles did not pick a 'plain Jane' for his future Queen, and the Princess of Wales serves as an international symbol of what a woman without much influence or ability of her own can achieve in the mating stakes, providing she has 'cover girl' looks.

And all this is in spite of women's liberation and the feminist movement!

It is significant that the leaders of the women's movement tried to deny their femininity by burning their bras, donning unflattering dungarees and abandoning make-up, perfume or any of the other adornments traditionally worn by women to attract males.

Yet, these ardent feminists remain a minority. Younger women capitalize on the gains they have made, take the better jobs and shun marriage for many years, but most still like to look good, wear stunning clothes and, in the end, attract the best mate they can possibly find.

Despite women's advances in all walks of life, they are still, unlike men, expected to look gorgeous, as well as to excel in everything else. Thus, while male newsreaders are expected to be authoritative but can be downright ugly, their female colleagues are expected to be very good-looking with come-to-bed eyes and a sexy or girlish hint to their vocal performance. They are inched out of the job at the first sign of less-than-youthful looks while the men are allowed to carry on — wrinkles and all.

MEN'S VIEWS OF MAKE-UP

In 1986, Vichy, the French cosmetics company, did some research in which they showed pictures of the same model with and without make-up to hundreds of men, picked at random. Sixty seven per cent chose the version in which she wore hardly any make-up, a glowing skin and a casual hairstyle; the higher their class and education, the higher this 'look' rated. Of those men who preferred the girl with a lot of make-up and a dyed and permed hairstyle (a smaller over-all number) most were of lower educational and class backgrounds.

According to American research, the less confident a man or woman feels, the more perfume/toiletries/make-up they use. Also, the more educated they are, the more self-assured they feel and the less they use those things.

CHAPTER THREE

THE ECONOMICS OF COSMETICS

THE REAL COST OF COSMETICS

The ingredients in a jar or tube or bottle of cosmetics perfume or toiletries invariably cost less than their packaging, and substantially less than the cost of selling them to us, the consumers.

According to figures produced in America, only about 25 per cent of every dollar spent — at most — is spent on the actual ingredients, labour and production costs of the product itself. The remaining three-quarters of the final cost are spent on advertising (approximately 10 per cent on average, but much more for launches) with nearly half going on retail distribution, including the profits made by the shop actually selling the stuff.

This explains why manufacturers are able to sell their products to staff employees for a few pence, when the same products are sold in the shops for several pounds. Charles of the Ritz, for example, charges employees 25p for lipsticks selling in the shops for £7 and the same for nail varnishes selling for over £5. Employees pay only 50p for sparkling rainbow eye shadow palettes which sell for £9 each.

In contrast, it also suggests that companies who are less generous to staff, like Avon, who knock only a third off the normal retail price, are not exactly losing out. Indeed, as they are not paying delivery or sales commissions on top, they are quite possibly making as much selling to staff as they do by selling to people outside the company.

It also explains why cosmetics companies are so generous with free samples to beauty editors. It is because the actual products cost them very little. They amount to a bribe when you consider the benefits to them of free publicity in the editorial columns.

A favourable mention in an editorial column is considered by the industry (and the media) to be worth about ten times any advertisement because the reader may believe that editorial endorsement denotes some sort of independent assessment (which almost certainly hasn't taken place), whereas it is clear that an advertisement placed by the company concerned is biased in favour of the product.

PROFITS AND PRICES

Cosmetics companies aim on average to make overall profits of the order of 15 to 20 per cent. Wholesale prices are roughly two thirds of the retail price which makes wholesale perfume prices, for example, much the same as the duty-free prices.

In 1980, Revlon, Shulton and Lanvin were all investigated by the Office of Fair Trading because of complaints that they were illegally forcing retailers to guarantee a minimum price at which they would sell their products. The practice had been abolished under the Resale Prices Act of 1976. After the inquiry all the companies promised that they would end their price-fixing activities and that retailers could sell their products at whatever price they considered fair.

The trade and financial press continue to report that the cosmetics industry is still one of the most profitable there is, in terms of return on investment. True, there were some lean years during the recession of the 1970s, but few companies collapsed and many thrived.

However, the business is volatile and customers are fickle and faddish, so some products make considerable profits, whilst others act as 'loss leaders'. Many of these are scrapped for purely commercial reasons, which can be very irritating to those customers who have got into the habit of using them. The 'own brand' companies, which are particularly liable to do this, include Marks and Spencer and Boots. They rely on vast turnovers to justify continuing each individual product and so, although they have a few consistent products, they tend to change whole lines from one season to the next.

THE RISE OF 'OWN BRANDS'

A recent trend has been the decision by most high street stores to sell their own brands of cosmetics. Marks and Spencers, Sainsbury's, British Home Stores, Next and Principles all do their own ranges at very competitive prices, even compared with those offered by Boots, the 'daddy' of them all, with more than a third of total cosmetics sales. Sainsbury's experimented at first with selling Revlon cosmetics, (as did Tescos, Key-Markets and Fine Fare). This went so well that Sainsbury's launched their own brand, *Natur*, followed by 'J' in 1981, which sells in 200 of their 270 stores.

We seem to like buying our face-creams and lipsticks with the cornflakes and soap-powder as about a quarter of all cosmetics and toiletries are now bought as own brands. In supermarkets, the 'no frills' approach of the large stores appeals to many women who are intimidated or irritated by conventional cosmetics saleswomen, and market analysts reckon that contrary to expectations this is the fastest growing section of the cosmetics industry. Indeed in 1979, a Boots spokesman, who must now be eating his words, confidently told a *Financial Times* writer that he doubted very much if cosmetics buyers would switch from buying in chemists to buying in supermarkets.

SELLING — THE MAKE-UP MERCHANTS

We all know them don't we? The heavily but immaculately made-up women behind the cosmetics and perfume counters — intimidatingly dressed, often in a uniform or scientific white coat.

Their 'Can I help you, Madam?' is often accompanied by, you suspect, a secret mouthing of, 'Lord knows you need it, you scruff.' Hot, bothered, already late for your next appointment, you either let them tell you what skin-cream is going to suit you or flee in shame, vowing next time to shop properly dressed, hair washed and cut, with at least a glimmer of confidence to be able to ask the right questions before parting with your cash or credit card.

You should always bear three things in mind. Firstly, these women are there to sell — not to offer a free consumer advice service — they may well be on commission. Secondly, their brief training will have filled their heads with prosaic words which they are obliged to repeat all day long. Thirdly, they are rarely independently trained as beauticians and so can tell you little other than the price of their goods and which size is the most economically priced.

Even when they swap companies, these women will still swear blind that whatever goods they are selling are the best available. If they do not, they are not doing their job — so don't expect impartial information.

We buy roughly a third of all our cosmetics and perfumes in department stores from saleswomen like these so it's worth bearing in mind what you are up against — if you hadn't already realized.

Occasionally, companies do employ independently trained beauticians and, if you have a particular problem, it is worth checking the assistant's credentials and asking to see 'the boss' rather than be fobbed off with someone who is merely selling the latest hype on commission.

FREEBIES — OFTEN BETTER THAN THE COSMETICS THEMSELVES

What the department store cosmetic counters offer, which the smaller outlets often don't, are the 'gift with purchase' goodies that often work out to be rather good value for the customer — certainly compared with buying the same items separately.

In fact, you may end up buying cosmetics, not for themselves, but for the gift. For example, Harrods one year offered a grey leather filofax for £25 if you bought some *Grey Flannel* product, and a towelling dressing gown free if you spent £15 on Dunhill goods.

This partly explains why so many people get lumbered with such brands at Christmas — we give them the toiletries, and keep the free goodies!

However, the industry has recently begun to realize what the customers are up to and have, in America at least,

started to baulk at such generous 'giveaways'. They have found that cosmetics customers now *expect* something free when they buy their products and often walk away after inquiring when the next 'special offer' is coming up. What began as a marketing gimmick is now a costly burden the industry would dearly love to dispense with. Few other industries give away such lavish presents when they sell their goods.

Estée Lauder, one of the companies at the forefront of this type of promotion, was the first to announce its policy of 'no more freebies' with its *Prescriptives* skincare line. The company's *Aramis* range has always been particularly Santa-like at Christmas-time and certainly made it difficult for rival companies to sell their products without presents. The industry has now realized that cosmetics customers are a fickle lot who will switch brands happily, providing the inducement to do so is right.

Hint
Try asking for free trial samples of new cosmetics and perfumes even if they aren't on display.

Some companies are also cutting back on the number of free trial samples they give away; most now keep such stocks under the counter and only the most enthusiastic and persistent of potential buyers receives them. Don't hesitate to ask for samples, especially of new cosmetics and perfumes. Skin-care samples often last for several applications and are very useful to carry around with you.

The shops which tend to get left out of this bonanza are those which are most accessible to most of us, but which for economic reasons offer the fewest bargains. These are the high street chemists, which cannot possibly compete and are gradually getting squeezed out by the chain stores and the department stores.

DIFFERENT COMPANIES — SAME PRODUCT

As far as the manufacturing process is concerned, most cosmetics companies do not make their own products from beginning to end, but contract the work out to suppliers of, say, essential oils, or packagers who merely put together the particular formula ordered. Thus certain shampoos and hair dyes, for example, are 'made' and marketed by different companies and appear to be very different but the ingredients are, in fact, identical.

ADVERTISING

The advertising of cosmetics, toiletries and perfumes forms a very large part of most countries' national advertising expenditure.

In America, individual agencies have turnovers which run into billions* of

*All references to 'billions' in this book are to the American billion i.e. one thousand millions.

dollars. In Britain, it is estimated that television alone scoops £5 billion a year from ads, a hefty proportion of which comes from the cosmetics companies. London Weekend Television, for example, charges £20,000 for each 30-second slot in non-guaranteed peak-time. Channel Four is cheaper, and is clogged with cosmetics ads, carefully timed to coincide with the kind of programmes the target market is likely to be watching — for example, hair gels and shampoos appear around the teenage pop programmes.

Full page ads in magazines aren't exactly cheap either. A page in a mass circulation weekly like *Woman*, with five million readers a week, costs £18,000 — many cosmetic companies prefer a more upmarket appeal in the monthly glossies which charge less. Even so, a full page colour ad in *Cosmopolitan* or *Good Housekeeping* costs over £5,000.

The perfume, toiletries, soap and drug companies spend proportionately more on advertising than any other industry.

Basically this is because we don't actually need the majority of the industry's products so we have to be forcefully persuaded that cosmetics are either indispensable or desirable.

The lavishness of the launches to alert the media to a new product have to be seen to be believed. Cosmetic and perfume companies think nothing of flying beauty editors half way round the world to lunch or to stay at top hotels while they ply them with champagne, glossy literature and free samples.

In 1977, Helena Rubinstein spent $3 million worldwide on launching their new 'Silk' make-up range. This included a lavish $350,000 launch on the shores of Lake Como, where a model rode around the spotlighted grounds of a luxury villa on a white horse. The irony was that make up using silk wasn't even a new idea, but one that had been around for years.

We, the consumers, have, of course, to pay for all this extravagance because the price of the product reflects this expenditure on launches.

PUBLICITY DISGUISED AS EDITORIAL MATTER

The public relations industry does very well out of the cosmetics companies and they serve easily digestible cheap editorial fodder to the magazines, many of which operate on tight budgets. Week after week, gorgeous free photographs

— in stunning colours or superb black and white — of pretty models wearing new products land on beauty editors' desks attached to blurbs written by the PR people. Often these photos and their captions appear unedited in the magazines as virtually unpaid ads, masquerading as independent editorial copy.

It is much cheaper for a magazine to use this PR material rather than to pay a photographer, model and journalist to supply a similar 'story'. This is partly why so much so-called 'beauty' editorial is merely publicity for new products.

Some companies even have the beauty editors on their payroll. One of the leading beauty editors from one of Britain's glossiest magazines was recently reported to have been recruited by a major cosmetics company as a consultant for the not inconsiderable annual fee of £500,000. Since MPs have to register their interests, perhaps beauty editors should be required to add a footnote to some of their features, mentioning if they are on a particular company's payroll?

Cosmetic companies quickly put magazines which don't toe the line in their place. Carol Sarler, feminist ex-editor of the now defunct *Honey* magazine tells how £20,000 of advertising was withdrawn the day after she was quoted in a national newspaper as saying she found it hard to show women looking intelligent when they were plastered with make up. It is surprising that she actually published four issues featuring bare-faced cover-girls before the industry took action. History now suggests that this was the ultimate sin for a women's magazine!

MILLION-POUND BUDGETS

On top of all this, million-pound advertising budgets for new products have become so commonplace that they are hardly worth noting as far as the industry is concerned.

Consumers might be surprised to know how much money is devoted to drawing their attention to cosmetics, etc. This is not merely for expensive perfumes, but also for quite ordinary things like suntan lotions, where an advertising budget of £500,000 a year is normal. Even re-launches have not insignificant budgets — *Femfresh*, a feminine hygiene product of the kind of which doctors disapprove and most people regard as highly inessential, was re-launched recently with a £250,000 advertising budget.

A chief executive of Ayer Barker advertising agency which handles ads for Chanel, Avon and Goya, among others, says cosmetics ads have to differ from others because their appeal is so ephemeral:

> If you are trying to sell fish fingers, you can stress the fact that your fish fingers contain 100 per cent cod. But people don't buy Chanel perfume because of what's in it. I don't think Chanel has ever said exactly what the ingredients of its perfumes are.

Pick up any glossy women's magazines and count the beauty ads. In the expensive journals like *Vogue* and *Harpers*, they account for nearly half the weight and actual content. There is a large amount of copycat advertising — so much so that, after 'scent-strips' first caught on, (instigated by *Giorgio* in 1982) magazines had to limit advertisers to two strips per issue because customers began to complain about the overwhelming smell of their magazines.

The next clever idea was three-dimensional advertising, using actual samples of powder to illustrate new lips and eye colours. Charles of the Ritz started it. Christian Dior followed and soon other companies were doing the same thing, even though these ads cost considerably more than conventional advertising.

Cosmetics ads have one thing in common — the consumer is being persuaded that if only he or she buys the advertised products, material success — epitomized by furs, jewellery, prestige cars, handsome escorts — will all be theirs for the asking. They may not kid themselves that they can look like the models in the ads or on the magazine covers, but they want to imitate the lifestyle so badly that they fall for the bait and buy the product and dream a little each time they use it.

It was calculated by *Advertising Age*, the industry's 'bible', that in 1982, $26 million was spent on advertising *Oil of Ulay*. An incredible figure, but hardly surprising in view of the number of times a day Twiggy popped up on our television screens to extol the product's virtues! This particular product made a point of being secret about whatever magic ingredient it was that made it superior to all its rivals. Others go out of their way to identify some usually unique and scientific-sounding formula which gives their's the superior edge.

Twiggy, incidentally, let slip one of the cosmetics advertising industry's trade secrets, which is that the make-up said to be worn by the model is not necessarily what is used. Instead, whatever the make-up girl chooses, or even whatever the model herself has in her bag, is used in preference with perhaps a cursory smear of the 'new' product on top to justify the descriptive copy.

In response to the massive *Oil of Ulay* advertising spree, rival Almay handed over $13 million to Saatchi and Saatchi the following year to try and increase its share of the market.

REFLECTING THE TIMES

The advertising industry both reflects and helps to shape the image of the times. For instance, in the 1950s, the growing emancipation of women meant that they were less susceptible to the 'devices to attract and seduce a man' approach that had appealed before.

Advertisers began to make their copy more subtle, emphasizing that it was okay to be both feminine and ambitious and to want something more than the traditional women's interests.

Then, during the permissive 1960s, the advertising became more sexually direct and provocative. Billboard ads for cosmetics for example, showed lipsticks fully extended in their cases in a blatantly phallic form, designed to appeal to the girl who was not afraid of anything — least of all men.

Ads for Revlon's stunningly successful *Charlie* perhaps epitomized the liberated young woman of the time, sexually and economically free yet also sexy,

wearing make-up and smelling divine. The image had enormous impact and the marketing of *Charlie* turned the perfume industry upside down.

With *Charlie*, Revlon found a gap in the market. Previously, fragrance had divided clearly into two types — the cheap (and fairly nasty) and the expensive (usually French) perfumes. *Charlie* captured the middle ground and was followed by many imitators, e.g. Coty's *Smitty* and later scents like Max Factor's *Le Jardin*.

During the 1970s and 1980s, advertisers became acutely aware of the more demanding, consumerist attitude of buyers of cosmetics. This, together with the health and fitness boom, is reflected in their copy with the heavy use of impressive-sounding scientific 'proof' that their products are superior and, above all, necessary, for today's successful go-getting men and women.

THE 'PURE AND SIMPLE' BOOM

These days, we are constantly being reassured of the purity of a product by the *absence* of certain (by implication 'bad') ingredients i.e. implying that rival products still contain greasiness, allergens, chemicals or whatever. It is sur-

prising how many allegedly 'natural' cosmetics actually contain preservatives and artificial ingredients, but the research shows that customers believe 'natural' products to be superior to other products.

Strawberry shampoos, orange blossom conditioners, cucumber cleansers, apricot scrubs and herbal bath oils, etc., all have a powerful appeal to the discerning health-conscious 1980s purchaser, yet, if you look at the containers these come in, there is often nothing to indicate, apart from the name itself, what is actually in, or not in, the product itself.

Where such products are advertised, the advertisers are careful to keep the image as 'pure' and 'natural' as they can, thus a virginal blonde walks through fields of long grass or sunlit woods, to advertise a gentle brand of shampoo like *Timotei* or *Sunsilk*. However, the industry has been surprised by the reaction to their advertising. Research carried out by Heather Mulholland and Mark Harrison in 1988 found that both men and women found the blonde woman in the *Timotei* ads 'too perfect'. Both sexes revealed that they liked models to look realistic, *not* virginal, haughty or, at the other extreme, too sexy.

The researchers, who presented their unexpected findings to the Market Research Society's annual conference in Brighton, said that people found the ads for Calvin Klein's perfume *Obsession* 'too explicit' and that women felt it was dehumanizing, turning women into sex-objects by not showing the female's face.

Calvin Klein's $7 million TV commercials for *Obsession* were so provocative that America's Moral Majority were outraged by the original TV promotion and led a national outcry against such blatant portrayal of sexual freedom and exuberance. The ads, which suggested passionate sex but not promiscuity, featured a nude model, as the object of desire of three different men. The ads were deemed offensive and unacceptable by the British Advertising Standards Authority, and the Independent Broadcasting Authority and so were not shown here.

The wording in cosmetics ads is interesting, conveying the impression that products do things they actually do not. Phrases like 'help to fight' or 'promotes' or 'activities' or 'stimulates' or 'improves' are all very hard to prove or disprove.

In the late 1980s the cosmetics industry ads have been designed to appeal to women by showing men in sexually erotic poses, with the women in the photos as willing accomplices rather than the passive dolly-birds of years gone by.

APPROPRIATE SPONSORSHIPS

As we'll explore in Chapter 15 companies marketing men's products not only use sporting images to promote the macho appeal, but also sponsor sporting events from tennis to snooker, badminton and football to underline the 'fitness' ingredient of their goods, illusory as that may be. Some women's lines do the same thing — for example, Avon once sponsored the London Marathon.

Recognizing the likely interest of its market, Johnson and Johnson, the makers of *Empathy*, the hair-care range for the over 40s, sponsor bridge tournaments. The company was quite open about it, saying, 'Over four million people play bridge in the UK and many of these are women. By sponsoring this new Ladies' Pairs Championship we are hoping to increase awareness of the *Empathy* range amongst our target consumers . . .' At the other extreme, advertisers still try to persuade us all that to look *young*, as well as beautiful, is everything. Researchers in America recently studied this emphasis in some depth by monitoring cosmetics ads in *Vogue*, *Ms*, *Playboy*, *Women's Home Journal* and *Time*, throughout the 1960s and 1970s.

They found that although only 27 per cent of American women were aged under 30, 77 per cent of the ads promoting cosmetics and perfumes portrayed women under 30. At the same time, only 4 per cent of the ads depicted women who looked over 40, although 57 per cent of the female population were in that age-group.

CHAPTER FOUR

THE COMPANIES

The cosmetics industry is a very big business indeed. L'Oréal, the world's second largest company, is France's third biggest corporation, whilst Avon, which would hardly figure on any British person's list of top companies is, in fact, the largest cosmetics company in the world.

Several cosmetics companies have sales in excess of a billion dollars a year, whilst pharmaceutical companies like Eli Lilly, Bristol Myers, Gillette, Hoechst, Squibb and Proctor and Gamble still make hundreds of millions of pounds from worldwide sales of their cosmetics products.

Most buyers of cosmetics and perfume would probably be surprised to know that despite the designer names and famous brand images, such as Elizabeth Arden, most of the top cosmetics brands are now owned by corporations with diverse and often unglamorous corporate interests not commonly associated with beauty. Few companies still belong to the family in whose name they sell; Elizabeth Arden, Clarins and Nina Ricci being just a few of such names which come to mind. Of the great names in the industry, Estée Lauder is the only one still alive, and still has a firm hand in the vast company which operates under her name.

Many of the other famous name companies have been carved up, sold off and resold and merged during the 1970s, when every major pharmaceutical corporation seemed to want a slice of the cosmetics or perfume market. The ownership of some of the best-known names is the cosmetics industry is shown in the box.

WHO OWNS WHOM*

Almay belongs to Beatrice, a huge American food company.

British American Tobacco (BAT Industries) owns Cyclax, Morny, Lentheric and Yardley.

Beechams owns *Jovan* and *Silvikrin* (and until 1986, Germaine Monteuil).

Balenciaga and *Madam Rochas* perfumes belong to German pharmaceutical company Hoechst.

Coty belongs to Pfizer.

Clairol belongs to Bristol-Myers.

Charles of the Ritz belongs to Yves St Laurent.

Chesebrough-Pond belongs to Unilever.

Elizabeth Arden belongs to Eli Lilly.

Goya belongs to ICI.

Maybelline and *Coppertone* belong to Schering-Plough.

Helena Rubinstein belonged to Colgate Palmolive, and is now owned by Albi Enterprises.

Max Factor, Revlon and Mary Quant belong to Pantry Pride. Shulton (*Old Spice*) and Breck belong to American Cyanamid.

Vanderbilt and Ralph Lauren are owned by L'Oréal.

*Accurate at time of going to press

Recent takeovers include Max Factor, which was bought by the gigantic Revlon corporation at the end of 1986 for a staggering 345 million dollars. The acquisition means that Revlon now owns previously 'rival' brands such as *Maxi, Colorfast, Swedish Formula, Miners, Mary Quant* and *Outdoor Girl*, along with its own vast range of names. Not surprisingly the group (which is part of Pantry Pride) is now ranked the largest in Europe in the colour cosmetics market.

Several of the major cosmetics companies scrambled to try and buy the upmarket Charles of the Ritz group when the pharmaceutical company Squibb recently decided to sell it. The winner was the Yves St Laurent group, which paid a massive $630 million. These sums seem awesome but are perhaps not so extravagant when you consider that the public spent $432 million on Charles of the Ritz products in 1986.

Even these sums are eclipsed by the sale of Chesebrough-Pond, which owns *Vaseline Intensive Care* and all the *Ponds* cold cream range, for a huge 3.1 billion dollars.

COMPANY LEADERS

Just as the oil industry is dominated by a few giants, so the cosmetics industry is headed by an oligopoly and in each section of the industry there is a clear company (not 'brand') leader. For example, Pantry Pride (Revlon, Max Factor) now dominates the eye make-up market, Schering-Plough (*Coppertone*), the suntanning market and Bristol Myers (*Clairol*) the hair-colouring market.

Because of this domination, the prices of such goods are fixed by the leading company and lack of realistic competition means the consumer has to pay whatever price the 'top dog' believes to be possible. With the economies of large-scale production to hand, and, as we have seen, the fact that the ingredients themselves cost very little, this gives the leading companies enormous power to fix the price at whim.

As there are so many potential customers, companies like Revlon diversify their products to suit all types of consumer and all sizes of wallet. Their seven different brands include the up-market *Princess Marcella Borghese*, *Ultima II*, *Etherea* and *Fine Fragrance*, and the cheaper *Charlie*, *Natural Wonder*, *Revlon*, *Moondrops* and *Revlon Toiletries*. Often there is very little difference between these products, but they are marketed to give them different images and in different price ranges so the customer can choose what she perceives as 'her' type of product.

CUT-PRICE COSMETICS

A recent development in selling cosmetics is the emergence of companies who advertise a range of cosmetics from established companies for sale directly to the customers at a fraction of the price.

For example, Northdown Cosmetics, a Kent company, sells top name fragrances like Carven, Houbigant, Helena Rubinstein, Hardy Amies and Rochas for often only 25 per cent of the normal store prices. It is obviously worth looking for these ads, which appear in specialist magazines like the nursing press, rather than the mainstream ones.

Some cosmetics companies advertise a mail-order service directly to the public — sometimes offering a special deal, but usually not. Also, stores like Harrods take out full-page ads, especially before Christmas, for their special promotions. Since they often charge extra for postage and packing, these do not seem like a particularly good deal, unless you live in a remote part of the country where mail order is the only option if you want to buy these things.

DIRECT SELLING: AVON

What brand of cosmetics is never sold in shops yet is the biggest selling range not only in Britain but also anywhere in the world? The answer, of course, is Avon. The name that is so synonymous with the sound of suburban door chimes that American executives often refer to their sales-reps as 'ding-dongs'.

There are more than 1.4 million Avon representatives working around the world (100,000 in Britain) each selling more than seven hundred products exclusively on a direct-selling door-to-door basis, within their own specially defined area. Many of this unsalaried self-employed workforce earn a fraction of the salaries of their rivals who work in high street stores all around the country.

Avon's approach has resulted in phenomenal sales — a *third* of all make-up used by British women is made by Avon. That means that of the 18 million women who wear lipstick six million regularly use one made by Avon! Similarly, of the six out of ten women who wear eye make-up, two out of ten regularly use Avon products, while of the three million women who use a blusher, almost half buy their compacts from Avon reps.

In 1986, Avon celebrated its centenary, and the company of the 1980s, with its new 'up-market' ranges, is very different to its 1960s predecessor with its overwhelmingly suburban image.

FROM BIBLES TO PERFUME

The Avon cosmetics company started in America almost by accident. Its founder, David McConnell, a bookseller, started giving away small sample bottles of perfume to each customer who purchased a bible. He quickly discovered that even his evangelical customers preferred the contents of the bottles to the bibles themselves, and so he decided to expand the cosmetics side of his business. At first, he concentrated on the perfume business, and by 1897 had recruited more than 100 members of staff for his warehouse in New York and about 10,000 agents selling direct to over a million customers.

At that time, the California Perfume Company, as it was known, presented no threat to the existing American cosmetics selling in stores because it was reaching people in remote places who would not otherwise have purchased, or even known about, such products. His business went from strength to strength and in 1939 he changed its name to Avon, calling it after the birth place of Shakespeare, whom he greatly admired.

In 1959, Avon came to Britain — its first and most important European outpost. Nearly 30 years later, its European headquarters at Northampton are so vast that entire lines for export to the rest of Europe and other parts of the world are produced there. Within seven years of its obscure arrival in the UK, Avon had become one of the top four cosmetics companies and a household name, even if not every household contained its products.

PHENOMENAL GROWTH

The growth in world sales has been almost unbelievable. Even in 1960, sales topped $168 million, and had doubled to $352 million five years later, and doubled again to $759 million in 1970. In 1972, it topped the billion dollar sales mark, and by 1977 it had sales worth a staggering $1.85 billion. Profits dropped dramatically in 1974 and 1975 and then picked up again.

The rapid increases that had characterized the last twenty years, slowed down by the 1980s, but even so, in 1983, Avon had passed the $3 billion mark in terms of annual sales.

Avon's worst time was in 1974, when people stopped buying the rather fancy packages and relatively expensive gift items that were just totally out of place in those economically depressed times. Financial analysts reckoned that Avon executives had got so used to the money never running out that they had lost touch with reality.

An expenses purge began; the executives stopped flying round the world first class. Advertising, which had dwindled to less than $7 million a year, was quadrupled, mainly to recruit new Avon ladies, and in America, incentive prizes were made more glamorous to encourage sales. Although the results of this all quickly paid off in terms of a return to high profits, it proved, for the first time, that even Avon Cosmetics was not recession-proof.

COLLECTORS ITEMS

An unexpected side-effect of the lean years was the discovery that many of the Avon perfume bottles had become collectors' items. This is because the moulds are broken after the factory run has been completed and so they acquire a rarity value once they can no longer be bought new. Some old glass and ceramic containers are now worth hundreds of pounds, and there are more than a hundred Avon collector's clubs in America.

Although Avon products have never and will never be sold retail, the company did try to set up its own Avon beauty salons in the 1970s. They pulled out when they realized that the customers were not coming back and the company lost $6 million over seven years in the attempt to make its products even more readily available.

These days, the British Avon plant has become so economically crucial in their multinational set up, that, in 1986, it was found to be more cost-effective to manufacture the exclusive and very expensive new *Deneuve* perfume at Northampton, and then export it solely for the American market. You could not buy it in Britain.

AVON IN BRITAIN

The Northampton plant has buildings and warehouses the size of airport hangers. On one floor there are enormous vats of body lotions, aftershaves and mascara, and kegs of powder. These are pumped to the floor below and carefully measured into the right containers on the production line, where they are weighed, packaged and boxed. The same powder is used in talcum powder as in face and eye-shadow powder and this is imported from Spain and Italy.

There are also laboratories where checks are regularly taken for any signs of bacterial contamination, and, when I visited in September 1986, the company prided itself on not having had such an outbreak in more than 18 months.

However, there have been some unfortunate episodes. For example, in 1971, Avon made the headlines in America when nearly 15,000 tins of baby powder had to be recalled because a pneumonia-type bacteria had somehow got into a batch. The company had to recall a batch of one of its night creams when bacteria was discovered by the ever-vigilant US Food and Drugs Administration, in the same year.

Ten years after the company first arrived in Britain, demand was such that a new computer centre was built at Corby, where 500 staff deal with between 7,000 and 8,000 orders every day. Each representative is guaranteed that orders will be filled within seven days and delivered to customers before they have changed their minds, or been tempted to buy their goods in the shops instead.

THE AVON REPS

The Avon reps collect 30 per cent commission on anything they sell. They start by buying a basic kit of samples in an Avon shopping bag and are given a 'territory', which is usually no more than two hundred homes, in the area in which they live.

The 100,000 reps are left almost entirely alone to make what they want to of their pitch. Many reps only sell to their immediate family and friends, some even buy merely for themselves. But if another 'pushier' rep comes along for the same area, Avon will move the smaller operator aside and persuade her to become a 'customer' of her more aggressive successor instead.

The British Avon company is reticent

about how much its reps can and do earn. According to American research, few Avon reps earn the Federal minimum wage and most earn little more than $2 an hour, especially if you take into account their travelling time and their expenditure on the telephone, postage, stationery etc.

The reps buy the products at 30 per cent of the brochure price, and the 30 per cent mark-up is their profit on each item. They can also buy products for themselves at this price, as can all other members of the company's staff. In addition, they can buy 'lucky bags' for £1 each, which contain about £14 worth of goods at normal prices, most of which are discontinued lines or ones which are not selling well.

In America, it is reckoned that about half the reps quit each year, to be replaced with others eager to take over. British statistics can only be guessed at, since the company does not release details.

CUSTOMERS NOT AT HOME

Avon's strength has always been in the 'mass market', in the working and lower middle classes. Because its unique selling method was directed towards women at home, its products tended to be brought mostly by housewives or young mothers. By the mid-1970s, Avon had run into difficulties because the recession had forced many more women out to work, and when the Avon lady called, they simply weren't at home. Since then, there has been a concerted attempt to reach women at work, by recruiting reps who work in offices. In 1986, Avon's American president told a meeting of cosmetics industry heads that 25 per cent of Avon sales were made to women at work and 50 per cent of its customers now had jobs, as opposed to being housewives.

GOING UPMARKET

Avon's UK President and Chief Executive, Paul Southworth, who was appointed in 1984, saw one of his principle objectives as persuading middle class and career women to buy his products, and many new 'up-market' lines were deliberately introduced.

The Junior Health Minister, Conservative MP for Derbyshire South, Mrs Edwina Currie, is the sort of 'up-market' client Avon likes to catch and keep. She buys Avon because she never gets time to shop for things like cosmetics. 'When you're working 14 hours a day there's not a lot of time left,' she told *Woman* magazine in 1986.

More surprisingly, she revealed that the Avon 'lady' she uses is in fact a policeman at the House of Commons, who tucks the latest brochures behind a statue of Disraeli. 'We often discuss moisturizers and he's a real expert on handcream,' she added.

AVON'S RIVALS

Avon considers its rivals to be the shops selling retail, not the other direct selling companies like Mary Kay, Oriflame or even the Universal Beauty Club. True, Avon's and Boots' own brands together probably account for the majority of all cosmetics and toiletries bought. However, there is still a significant market for the other direct-selling companies, each of whom has a slightly different sales technique.

ORIFLAME

Oriflame is a Swedish company whose biggest market is, in fact, the UK. In 1985 it sold nearly £40 million worth of products, making a £5.9 million profit, and its 1986 profits are believed to have increased by another 12 per cent. Because you do not see their products in the shops (indeed, you may never have heard of them) you may assume that this is a small operation. In fact, according to the company's figures, *Oriflame* is the third or fourth largest selling skin-care range in the UK.

Its sales-force consists of 3,800 consultants in the UK, who sell their products through demonstrations or 'dems' as they are known in the company. Each consultant makes sales worth between £14 to £20 per demonstration, with the average customer ordering £9.31 worth of cosmetics. Most aim to demonstrate at three parties a week, which can give them up to £60, before taking into account their overheads, like the telephone and travel. The commission on every sale is worth 23.5 per cent, but it rises by another 7.5 per cent if sales exceed £375 a month. The basic sales kit costs £45 but its retail value is about £170.

The demonstrations are organized with the help of a friend, called the 'hostess', who is given a small gift which is carefully valued on a sliding scale, according to how much is sold. She also gets a free facial, and by agreeing to provide the setting for the demonstration, she also volunteers to be the model on which the skin care and make-up is demonstrated by the consultant.

Skin care line is the biggest selling range of products sold by Oriflame, and costs about £20 for a basic set. The make-up also sells well, accounting for nearly as much as the skin care, while a very small proportion of sales involve men's products and fragrances.

Oriflame consultants think they are nothing like Avon reps, whom they see as little more than saleswomen who make very little money. Oriflame women who do particularly well become group managers and then earn a percentage on the sales of all consultants working in their groups as well as 31 per cent on all their own sales. The company insists that such women (who, like their Avon counterparts, are still unsalaried and survive solely on their percentages), can make a career rather than merely a part-time job out of their activities.

Unlike Avon, Oriflame does not have a large number of black customers, although some black women do like their colour make-up (eye shadow, lipstick, etc.). The company did investigate the possibility of bringing out a special black make-up line but decided that it would not be very successful.

One problem Oriflame has is that it 'loses' customers because people buy at a demonstration and they may never go to another one again, and there is no other straightforward way of contacting the Oriflame consultant. Because of this, the company has recently launched a mail-order Beauty Club. Members receive details of products six times a year and can buy at a 25 per cent discount. The consultants who originally introduced them also get a percentage on their purchases. The goods the club members buy are mailed directly to their homes.

MARY KAY COSMETICS

Mary Kay is a household name in America. Mary Kay Ash has built a cosmetics empire from nine saleswomen in 1963 to a 200,000 sales force with total sales worth more than $300 million a year.

Mary Kay Ash's favourite colour is pink — bright pink — and there are now more than 750 pink Mary Kay Cadillacs driven around America by her prize-winning mega-selling top salesmen and saleswomen. Other prizes her best employees can win include diamond rings, fur coats, diamond-encrusted pins shaped like bumble-bees and Oldsmobiles for those who do not get as far as winning the prized pink Cadillacs.

It is a totally American, approach which obviously appeals to Americans and does extremely well for all concerned. But, when Mary Kay came to 'open England' she was astonished and disappointed at what she found. Providing her consultants with a case of goodies and sending them out to sell, sell, sell, just wasn't that easy.

She said in an interview in the *Washington Post* in 1984,

> One of the things that surprised me to pieces was, over here [in the USA] if a girl wants to become a consultant you just say 'that's wonderful! Here's the agreement, the case is $85 and let's get started.' Over there, I have to wait seven days before I take your cheque — a cooling-off period they call it. Well, in seven days, your husband or your mother-in-law can talk you out of it. And really, it's dangerous... You know, women are impetuous, and some of the best decisions I've ever made were the impetuous ones. I knew it was right and I did it. But if I'd had seven days to think about it...

In fact, Mary Kay was a disastrous flop in the UK. During its short-lived time in Britain it is thought by the cosmetics industry to have lost over £1 million. Sales continued to be so disappointing that in December 1986 it pulled out of Britain altogether and Mary Kay returned to Dallas licking her wounds.

AMWAY

Amway is another company which is a huge success in America in the direct selling business but which has yet to make a significant impact on cometics buyers in Britain. However, with a base in Milton Keynes and a growing number of door-to-door sales people, it could grow bigger. Amway also offers household goods, and nutritional products as well as cosmetics.

YVES ROCHER

This is a French company which has a few retail outlets but which sells most of its products by mail order. They are not cheap, but the company runs a series of promotions designed to encourage customers to buy more.

Skin care is a speciality. Most of the 400 items in the range are made from 'natural' ingredients, manufactured in France.

OTHER MAIL-ORDER COSMETICS COMPANIES

There are some companies which specialize in buying from various manufacturers at a discount and then selling the goods to members at a bargain price. They are an excellent way of experimenting with a selection of products you might not otherwise try or discover for yourself, especially if you do not have access to shops selling the latest and widest selection of cosmetics and toiletries. The snag is that you may end up sometimes buying 'blind' products which are useless to you.

The cosmetics companies co-operate because by selling their products — albeit at a discount — through these clubs, and they are reaching potential customers they might otherwise not win and who might continue to buy their products on a regular basis, after sampling them first.

UNIVERSAL BEAUTY CLUB

The best known of these companies is probably the Universal Beauty Club. This was started by Doreen Miller, who still keeps a firm hand on the company, even though it is now international and has more than 120,000 members in Britain alone.

Every six to eight weeks members receive a box of six make up, skin care or perfume products worth about £12 retail, for which they pay £5 plus postage. The introductory kit is sold at a further discount.

The snag is that members only get the chance to reject the latest kit when they have opened it, and returning it means a trip to the Post Office, postage costs and hassle so that members usually find it easier to keep the kit, even if they don't want the goods. But, unlike mail-order book and record clubs, membership can be cancelled at any time as there is no minimum commitment.

'NEW YOU' BEAUTY PROGRAMME

This was started in 1980 by the Kingfisher Publishing Group, which like the UBC, publishes a booklet on beauty care and treatments. It is aimed at younger people who want to learn about make-up, and in its first year attracted over 100,000 teenage members. The packages cost £7 a month plus postage and VAT, which usually leaves little change out of ten pounds. They claim to be worth much more.

Many other cosmetics companies run mail-order lines and it is always worth asking about these especially if it is difficult for you to get to shops.

CHAPTER FIVE

COSMETICS IN OTHER COUNTRIES

THE EASTERN BLOC

Even countries behind the Iron Curtain such as USSR and China have cosmetics and toiletries industries — some of which are for export and the rest for home consumption.

Although cosmetics have been in use in China for more than 5,000 years, the perfume industry is only some 50 years old. With the increasing rise in the people's living standards, more and more are demanding perfumes and cosmetics as used and enjoyed in the West. With a wealth of traditional medical love, a rich variety of natural resources, and a cheap and inexhaustible labour force, the Chinese cosmetics industry is likely to grow and grow.

Already the toiletries sector is well developed and China produces, for example, 350 million tubes of medicated toothpaste a year — which supplies more than a third of the demand. (The rest of the population use a variety of tinctures made from ancient herbal remedies known to combat decay and halitosis. No doubt, some enterprising British cosmetics company will soon be pinching the formulas!)

Until about a decade ago, the authoritarian rule of the Chinese Communist Party meant that concern about physical appearance was considered vain and unacceptable, and sombre uniforms and no adornments were the order of the day. At the time of the Red Guard, any Chinese woman who wore dresses, make-up, or jewellery was persecuted.

However, in the more relaxed 1980s, China even has its own models, who enjoy much admiration internationally and super-stardom back home. They lead extraordinary lives compared to their contemporaries — renting apartments, owning televisions and stereos, wearing clothes and make-up and, above all, earning more than junior government ministers.

In 1985, China even held its first beauty contest sponsored by, among others, the Communist Youth League.

This was a unisex event in which ten men and ten women competed for the title. For most women, however, it is likely to be many years yet before they will be able to afford the sort of 'look' that the country's few top models now display to the world. When — and if — they are, there is a vast market for the cosmetics industry. As a sign of what's possibly to come, two of the world's biggest cosmetics companies, Avon and L'Oreal, are involved in the Chinese expansion, as are Wella and Nivea.

In the USSR and other Eastern Bloc countries, the current emphasis seems to be on health-related cleansing and skin care products rather than those purely designed for frivolous vanity. Mrs Raisa Gorbachev may well set the style with her fashionable and obviously carefully groomed appearance, and the signs are that no part of the world, whatever its regime and culture, is immune from the appeal of cosmetics.

JAPAN

Japan is quite different. Indeed, its two leading companies Shiseido and Kanebo, are both in the top five worldwide, mainly because of their sales among the Japanese.

One of the reasons for this, as British cosmetic industry barons often complain, is that the Japanese put up complicated trade barriers which either make it impossible to import cosmetics made by the rest of the world, or force up the prices so they are uncompetitive with home-produced cosmetics.

On the whole, the Japanese do not use perfume because they think that it may be used to disguise other unpleasant smells. However, the French, in particular, have been trying to prise open the door of the vast potential Japanese market in the knowledge that if they can, there are billions of francs to be made.

The size of the Japanese market is shown by the fact that in retail sales, the industry is worth three times the British industry — indeed, sales of cosmetics in Japan outstrip those of Britain, Germany and Italy combined, in terms of millions of dollars. Only Americans eclipse the Japanese for cosmetics purchases. Unlike the European markets, which have slackened in recent years, the Japanese market has grown at the rate of 15 to 20 per cent a year for the past two or three decades.

Since other countries do not put up trade barriers against Japan, a vast amount of her cosmetics are exported to both European countries and to America. This is backed by lavish advertising in the glossy magazines in all the

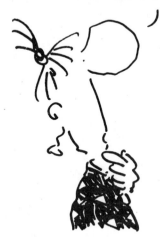
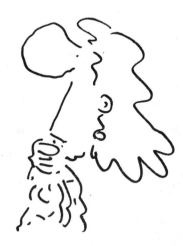

HMM! I WONDER WHAT COSMETICS ARE LIKE IN OTHER COUNTRIES?

countries. Informative brochures promoting Japanese products and showing how they should be used can be found on counter displays in stores like Harrods and Maceys.

The Japanese emphasize the uniqueness and the 'beauty secrets' of their ancient traditions, together with the efficiency of the country's production techniques.

Here is an example from Kanebo, promoting their *Silkbody* range, which costs approximately £10 a bottle for gel, bath essence, lotion, or scrub cream:

The line brings together the latest dermatological findings with all the tradition of the Japanese bathing ceremony, to bestow a feeling of well-being on both body and spirits.

(Whether any product has that power in an English bathroom as opposed to a Japanese spa is somewhat doubtful, but never mind, the prose sounds pretty.)

The top three Japanese companies are Shiseido, followed by Kanebo, with half its sales, and then Kao, with another half the volume again. Only two non-Japanese companies figure in the top 10, and they are Max Factor at 8 and Avon, at number 10, whilst Wella is the 12th biggest and Revlon limps behind at number 23, followed by Estée Lauder at 28th place.

There is a massive choice of sales outlets in Japan, with around 25,000 different points of sale, as well as a thriving mail order and door-to-door clientèle.

Although there is not a vast amount of money in some of the South-East Asian countries, the more affluent parts like Singapore and Hong Kong provide excellent export markets for the Japanese cosmetics industry.

MIDDLE EAST

In strict Muslim societies, perfume has always been one of the very few precious luxuries allowed — alcohol and other sinful habits like smoking having been strictly forbidden, especially to women. Perfume is an acceptable gift, even during the feast of Ramadan, when everyone fasts for a month.

Arab women with money to spare buy a great deal of perfume. They prefer the most expensive, musky, heavy scents, such as *Cartier, Giorgio, Opium, Magie Noire, Shalimar*, whilst Western expatriates favour the lighter perfumes like *Anaïs Anaïs*.

As a gesture towards the more restricted way of life, some of the more sexy ads used to advertise these perfumes are toned down for the Arab market so as not to offend the Muslim religious leaders, otherwise the perfume manufacturers could lose their licences to sell.

AUSTRALIA AND NEW ZEALAND

Australia and New Zealand have markets similar to those in Europe where all the big names in perfumes and cosmetics are readily available. Both the Australian and American Consumers' Associations have been particularly active in monitoring the activities of the cosmetics industry and in scrutinizing and analysing many different types of cosmetics, from hair transplant techniques to skin and hair care products.

The research is as thorough as you would expect from such organizations, and is significant enough to be reproduced in full in the glossy international cosmetics trade journals. For example, when the Australian Consumers' Association tested more than

100 different skin cleansing products in 1986, the journal *Cosmetic World News* devoted two full pages to their report, which 'quite a nasty shock for some of the top cosmetics companies.' Amongst those that fared badly in the tests were Estée Lauder, Avon, Revlon's *Ultima II* and *Nivea*, whilst a cleanser by Yves Rocher came out best in the trial.

Australia and New Zealand have many of their own cosmetics companies whose names are not known on the other side of the world, but which have a substantial following at home.

THE EUROPEAN COSMETICS MARKET

The cosmetics market in Europe is worth about $10 billion a year in sales of cosmetics and toiletries.

There is a greater emphasis on scientific skin care (especially in Scandinavia, France and West Germany) than there is in either Britain or America. Indeed, the preoccupation of the European industry is with health and maintenance of the skin and hair, and a natural look, rather than artifice.

The French are particularly body-conscious and often worry more about their beauty from the neck downwards rather than upwards. A whole industry has grown up around 'cellulite', the 'orange-peel' sort of skin that shows above where fat has lodged.

Klorane's *Elancyl*, which contains ivy and coffee plant extracts, is the only slimming and toning method of its type to have been awarded the Visa PP, issued by the French Ministry of Health for having proved itself to reduce adipose tissue. The tests claim that the *Elancyl* method can 'shrink' stubborn excess skin more than an inch in circumference in one month. Many experts believe that cellulite can be elimated by ordinary dieting and exercise regimes, and that massage with anything will tone the body. However, despite this, and the fact that many experts in Britain refuse to acknowledge that cellulite even exists, *Elancyl* has enormous worldwide sales and no significant rivals.

The French, or course, dominate the international perfume industry, mainly for historical reasons, but also because they happen to be very good at it and continue to develop perfumes that sell well all over the world. French perfume ads tend to use more naked bodies than ads elsewhere in the world, underlining the association between seductive smells and sex.

The French buy proportionately more

suncare products than other Europeans, being keen sunworshippers (and with *Ambre Solaire* they have one of the best-known brands). But they spend less on toiletries and hair care than the Germans who spend more on toiletries and cosmetics than any other European country, and there is particular growth in men's products and skin care. The lowest use of cosmetics is in Holland and Luxemburg, where increases in sales in recent years have barely kept pace with inflation. No-one really knows why the relatively affluent Dutch have not taken to cosmetics but it just hasn't happened. Its home-grown industry is very small and it remains to be seen whether the gigantic companies will one day manage to colonize the unaffected Dutch.

CHAPTER SIX

ANIMALS IN PERIL — THE UGLY SIDE OF THE BEAUTY BUSINESS

It is repugnant to many people that vast numbers of animals are used by the cosmetics and perfume industry both for safety testing and as actual ingredients in their products.

Whilst the use of animals for medical research may be tolerated, their role in cosmetics is more controversial. As a result, there is a sizeable chunk of the cosmetics industry which now sells products guaranteed not to have been produced at the expense of any animal.

TESTING COSMETICS ON ANIMALS

Cosmetics companies are obliged, through the consumer safety regulations, to test their products carefully before marketing them so as to minimize any risks of allergy and irritation — or worse — to humans.

Testing of cosmetics is required not only for conventional use — for example, to see if there is any long-term damage from swallowing small but repeated quantities of lipstick — but also for accidental contact, for example, by a child spraying itself in the face with an aerosol deodorant, eating a lipstick or painting its lips with nail varnish. These things may sound bizarre, but each year there are about 800 such accidents, although fatal poisoning from cosmetics is almost unheard of.

There are rare cases, like the schoolboy who accidentally killed himself in 1986 after inhaling fumes from an aerosol deodorant, but these come under the heading of 'solvent abuse' and there is little that any industry can do to protect itself from such tragedies.

However, by running the safety tests that the legislation requires of them, the cosmetics companies risk offending potential customers who happen to be animal lovers. The number of animals used in testing cosmetics and toiletries has actually been decreasing in recent years, halving from more than 30,000 in 1980 to just over 15,700 in 1986. This represents less than half of one per cent of the estimated 3 million animals used each year for vivisection and testing purposes by the medical, veterinary and pharmaceutical industry. Even so, these experiments are still controversial because their purpose is, to many people, essentially trivial. The most popular species used for testing are rats and mice, followed by rabbits and birds, then guinea pigs and fish.

The good news is that for the sixth successive year, there has been a six per cent drop in the number of animals used to test cosmetics. However, this is not because of a change of heart on the part of the industry, but rather that there is less testing to do — so many ingredients already being available, and also because the business of testing is very costly.

THE DRAIZE TEST

We do not need thousands of different shampoos and conditioners; old formulations — albeit in pretty new packaging — are preferred by many people if the alternative involves rows of rabbits being forced to have huge quantities of stinging chemicals poured into their eyes. This is routinely done in what is known as the Draize test, to see how much it takes to cause permanent damage.

You don't have to be an animal fanatic to appreciate how painful it must be if you consider how much it stings just to spill a drop of soap or shampoo in your eye. Over 150,000 rabbits are used each year, usually albinos because they have no tear ducts and so cannot cry and wash away the source of irritation.

In 1980, a powerful campaign started in America, the main targets being Revlon and Avon, the cosmetics industry's leaders, to persuade them to find some alternative to the Draize test. The campaign culminated in animal liberationists taking out large ads in the *New York Times*, showing a rabbit with sticking plaster over its eyes, asking people to stop buying Revlon's products unless they developed an alternative to the Draize test.

Unlike previous more direct approaches to the company, this one worked, and after demos outside Revlon's offices by people dressed in bunny costumes, Revlon announced it was donating $250,000 a year for three years to Rockefeller University to explore the alternatives. Avon followed suit, and so did Estée Lauder and some of the other leading companies.

It is possible that this has an effect on

the industry, because although there were over 7,000 Draize tests carried out on animals in Britain in 1986, this was 1,000 fewer than two years earlier, showing a substantial decrease, and Home Office figures show that this downward trend has been maintained for the last decade.

THE LETHAL DOSE TEST

The other test that upsets many people is the Lethal Dose (LD) 50 test, which is the one in which experimental animals are force-fed or plastered in enormous quantities of, say, bath gel or hand lotion, to see how much their intestines or skins can survive before *half* of them die. This period may last days or even weeks.

The LD 50 test has been seriously challenged by many scientists who doubt its usefulness, especially in cosmetics testing— after all, how many people are going to eat a mountain of lethal lipstick, or drink gallons of astringent? And what does it tell us about potential human poisoning if it takes x pints of anti-perspirant for a guinea pig to die?

MORE RIGHTS FOR ANIMALS

On a more official level, there have been a number of unsuccessful attempts, over the years, notably by peers in the House of Lords, to prohibit the use of animals in the testing of cosmetics. Although these have failed, new legislation was finally passed in 1986, after 10 years of negotiation in Home Office committees, that gave experimental animals more rights than they had hitherto enjoyed throughout the whole history of cosmetics industry.

These include the rule that before applying a substance to the eye in a Draize test, the laboratory technician concerned must be sure that a severe adverse or painful reaction could not already be predicted. In addition, substances known from skin studies to be corrosive or severely irritating must not be put into an animal's eyes, and any specific test should be carried out on a single animal at least 24 hours before applying it to others.

Animals have to be closely monitored, and, if severe ocular damage occurs, the rules require them to be humanely destroyed, whilst, if in pain, they can be given painkillers. Before the Animals (Scientific Procedures) Act became law, painkillers were not given, so suffering could be intense.

As well as all these safeguards, the technicians now have to be licensed and this licence can be revoked if the rules are flouted. At the moment, there are very few Home Office inspectors to oversee the new rules protecting animals from unnecessary pain and suffering but the climate has changed and it is likely that fewer and fewer animals will be used in this way by the industry in future.

The cosmetics world is primarily a faddish and fashionable one which needs new products in order to survive and make further profits and these products need to be tested. However, alternative forms of testing are available, and cosmetics companies should be at the forefront of those willing to abandon animal testing in favour of something just as effective, but more humane.

No doubt there will be continued calls for a complete ban on the use of animals for testing cosmetics and toiletries — as there has been recently in West Germany. However, since the industry is multinational, a ban in Britain would merely involve transferring the laboratories to, say, France or America, and would make little difference to the amount of animal suffering involved.

Only a worldwide ban, or a steady turning away from those companies which test on animals towards those which guarantee they do not experiment on animals, will ensure that this kind of suffering is discontinued in the pursuit of beauty-enhancing products.

CRUELTY-FREE BEAUTY

Several companies already offer 'cruelty-free' products, by which they mean they do not use any ingredients which have had to be tested on animals.

As the health awareness movement has grown so has the demand for cruelty-free products. Possibly it was the anti-fur campaigns run by the animal liberation movement which led to the realization that the cosmetics industry — another part of the world of glamour and beauty — has some nasty secrets.

Whatever the reason, the public, including buyers of cosmetics, have become more aware of the cruelty involved in bringing them a vast range of safe products.

Now there are more than thirty companies which operate a policy of not testing their cosmetics on animals, including famous names such as Innoxa, Lentheric, Morny and Yardley.

Yardley is among the smaller number of companies — a half dozen or so, including The Body Shop and Creighton Laboratories — who can also guarantee that their products do not contain any animal-derived ingredients (such as lanolin).

BEAUTY WITHOUT CRUELTY

Beauty Without Cruelty was the first company in the market, starting in 1963. It had the field more or less to itself for many years — the trend-setters of the 1960s were not particularly aware of animal welfare issues.

BWC uses lanolin and beeswax in some of its products but these are not harmfully produced from animals and, although lanolin was tested on animals for cosmetics purposes years ago, no fresh tests are required if established ingredients like these are used. For the most part, BWC uses vegetable ingredients rather than by-products of the meat industry and, although vegetable ingredients are generally more expensive than meat by-products, BWC has kept its prices at a competitive level.

The company is very popular with vegetarians, particularly as a percentage of its profits is regularly handed over, not to the shareholders, who receive no dividends, but to anti-vivisection groups which explore the alternatives to animal research.

PURE PLANT PRODUCTS

Pure Plant Products was started in Cheshire not long after BWC, but the range is only sold on a mail-order basis or in health food shops and is consequently less well known to the majority of cosmetic buyers (Look in your health food shop).

THE BODY SHOP

This is perhaps the best known of the cruelty-free companies, although it is likely that most customers are drawn by the 'naturalness' of the ingredients as much as the absence of animal testing. The range includes a huge selection of natural ingredients, from almonds to nettles, orchids and pineapple to Viennese chalk, in more than 300 different products, about half of which are made by the Body Shop company itself. The rest are made by suppliers who have to follow the 'non-animal testing' rule.

Since its modest beginnings in Brighton 10 years ago, the Body Shop has grown phenomenally, thanks to the direction of its founder Anita Roddick, and its shares have rocketed, to the delight of investors and the founder herself, who has become a multi-millionaire.

There are now more than 250 Body Shops in Britain and other countries, all run on a franchise basis. This means that the people who actually manage and run the shops are not making a fortune out of the products, although the company is making profits in excess of £3 million a year.

The Body Shop's policy is not to waste money on fancy packaging, and its products are sold in plain plastic containers. (However, as natural ingredients are more expensive than synthetic ones, the prices charged make the products seem quite expensive compared with ranges produced by companies like Yardley or Marks and Spencer.) A curiosity is that, while the company boasts it uses as much recycled packaging as it can, its plastic shampoo bottles, for example, are still not biodegradable. However, it claims to be the only cosmetics company actively looking for biodegradable containers.

There is a definite appeal in this type of packaging, and the kind of customer who only buys Body Shop products is probably the sort of person who wouldn't be seen dead buying any of the more conventional cosmetics and toiletries on sale in other shops.

The Body Shop offers a refill service which salves the consciences of those who also go to the trouble of re-cycling their newspapers and empty bottles. Refills are cheaper to encourage the customer to refill old containers rather than buy new ones each time. Other companies have offered a refill service for roll-on deodorants for some years.

The Body Shop claims to be the first company in the UK to use jojoba, a plant extract that substitutes a wax for the oil produced by sperm whales. The rest of the industry has followed this trend but whether the number of sperm whales which are killed has been reduced, or merely the jojoba harvest increased, is very hard to pinpoint. However, it is clearly a trend that animal-lovers should follow.

CREIGHTON LABORATORIES

This Sussex-based company makes a range of natural products, including some it supplies to The Body Shop. Others it markets under its own name, and yet others under the name of Crabtree and Evelyn. The products are all of similar quality and composition but the image and marketing are very different.

THE SECRET GARDEN

This relatively new company also sells products which have not been tested on animals. Because the products are entirely natural, using no cheaper synthetic ingredients, they are somewhat expensive, but their quality is superb, and like the Body Shop, the customer pays little extra for the packaging. Furthermore, one of the founding directors, David Hircock, is a qualified pharmacist and herbalist and is therefore able to compare the active ingredients of his own formulations with those of his rival companies.

Two animal liberation organizations have been particularly active in highlighting the trade and use of animals in the cosmetics industry. They are the British Union for the Abolition of Vivisection, which publishes a magazine *Choose Cruelty Free*, copies of which are available from its headquarters, 16a Crane Grove, London N7, and Animal Aid, which also publishes details of cosmetics companies which sell cruelty-free products. Animal Aid is at 7, Castle Street, Tonbridge, Kent TN9 1BH and both organizations welcome new members. Neither is associated with the food poisonings and terrorist activities of the more extreme animal liberation groups.

The following companies' names have been supplied by both organizations:

Alo Cosmetics, Unit 2, Industrial Estate, Cranleigh Gardens, Southall, Middlesex UB1 2B2

Barry M, Mail order address: Unit 1, Bitteracy Business Centre, Bitteracy Hill, Mill Hill East, London NW7 1BA

Beauty Without Cruelty, Mail order address: 37 Avebury Avenue, Tonbridge, Kent TN9 1TL

The Body Shop International, Hawthorn Road, Wick, Littlehampton, West Sussex BN17 7LR

Bright Eyes & Caurnie, c/o Save, 2 Thornton End, Holybourne, Alton, Hants

Camilla Hepper, Mail order address: Lion House, 20-28 Muspole Street, Norwich, Norfolk

Caurnie Soap Company, The Soaperie, Canal Street, Kirkintilloch, Scotland G66 1QZ

Chandore Perfume, 2 Ashtree Avenue, Mitcham, Surrey

Cherish Cosmetics, Jane Kendall, Western View, Sunny Bank, Great Longstone, nr Bakewell, Derbyshire DE4 1TL

Creighton Products, Water Lane, Storrington, Pullborough, Sussex

Cruelty Free Cosmetics, PO Box 32, Stevenage, Herts SG1 1JS

Culpeper Ltd, 9 Flask Walk, London NW3

Ecover, Full Moon, Charlton Court Farm, Mouse Lane, Steyning, West Sussex BN4 3DF

Faith Products, 52-56 Albion Road, Edinburgh

G R Lane Health Products Ltd, Sisson Road, Gloucester GL1 3QB

Good Nature, 42 High Street, Bidford on Avon, Warwickshire B50 4AA

Hagman Laboratories, Wendover House, Beaconsfield Road, Friern Barnet, London N11 3AB

Haircare & Beauty, Beauty House,

815B Trading Estate Road, Park Royal, London NW10

Henara (Hair Health) Ltd, Classic House, 174/180 Old Street, London EC1

Honesty Cosmetics, 33 Markham Road, Chesterfield, Derbyshire S40 1TA

Inter-Medics Ltd, 52 Walsworth Road, Hitchin, Herts

James Kimber, Harold Place, Hastings, East Sussex

Jane Howard Cosmetics Ltd, 8 Woodburn Drive, Chapeltown, Sheffield, S. Yorks S30 4YT

Janco Sales, 11 Seymour Road, Hampton Hill, Middlesex TW12 1DD

Lorna & Sunita, Tally Ho, Woodcock Hill, Harefield Rd, Rickmansworth, Herts

Martha Hill, Mail order address: The Old Vicarage, Laxton, nr Corby, Northants

Mayflower Beauty Products, Lyndhurst Oaks, The Fairway, Godalming, Surrey

Meadow Herbs Ltd, Cophill Place, Anna Valley, nr Andover, Hants

Natures Secrets, Unit 1, Six Ways, Barnards Green, Malvern, Worcs

Natural Beauty Products Ltd, Unit 5, Kingsway Bdgs, Bridgend Ind Est, Bridgend, Mid Glamorgan

Naturally Yours Cosmetics Ltd, Freepost, 7 Tudor Rd, Broadheath, Altrincham, Cheshire WA14 5BR

New Era Labs Ltd, 39 Wales Farm Road, London W3 6XH

Pecksniffs, 45-46 Meeting House Lane, Brighton, Sussex

Perry Charlse, Flora Place, Wadebridge, Cornwall

Plumpurrs Skin Care, 39 Coverdale Road, Sheffield S7 2DD

Power Health Products, 10 Central Avenue, Airfield Est, Pocklington, Yorks YO4 2NR

Pure Plant Products, 42 Sandy Lane, Irby, Wirral, Merseyside

Queen Cosmetics, 130 Wigmore Street, London W1H OAT

Reform Cosmetics, The House of Regency, 5 Kingsway Buildings, Bridgend Industrial Estate, Bridgend, Mid-Glamorgan CF31 3SD

Rita Shaw, 3 Juniper Court, 26 College Hill Road, Harrow Weald, Middlesex HA3 7HE

Romany Herb Products, 10 Central Ave, Airfield Estate, Pocklington, York YO4 2NR

Simply Herbal, Murdoch, Kingsway, Wilton, Wilts SP2 OAQ

Tiki Cosmetics, Sisson Road, Gloucester GL1 3QB

Weleda, Heanor Road, Ilkeston, Derbyshire

Winston, Mail order address: Illingworth Health Foods, York House, York Street, Bradford

Witchwood, Oldfield Road, Bickley, Kent BR1 2LE

Yin Yang Beauty Care, Abbey Chase, Bridge Road, Chertsey, Surrey

ANIMALS AS INGREDIENTS

Parts of some animals are highly prized as vital ingredients, especially as scents or fixatives in luxury perfumes. Animal products are supposed to resist evaporation much longer than any synthetic alternatives and so they are highly prized, especially by the luxury end of the perfume industry.

MUSK AND MUSK DEER

Some species like the musk deer have been hunted almost to extinction in the East because of their bodily secretions. The uncastrated male musk deer secretes one of the most valuable fluids in the world from its sexual glands. It is worth half its weight in gold; it was once worth three times its weight in gold, but it is now cheaper than it used to be because of the availability of synthetic substitutes.

Musk takes 30 days to mature in the sacs of the young male deer and is produced from about the age of twelve months onwards. The secretion is probably used by males to scent the urine and the fluid is red in colour with a sweet smell.

To obtain one kilo of musk, 40 adult males have to be slaughtered, and since they are caught in traps, females are also killed in the pursuit. So for every kilo of musk, more than 100 deer actually die in poachers' traps. It is almost impossible for perfumiers today to obtain pure musk because of its high value, and supplies tend to be adulterated oriental medicines. There is also a thriving industry based on its dubious reputation as an aphrodisiac.

In the perfume industry, natural musk has largely been replaced by about 300 synthetic compounds which smell of the real thing. Companies like Jovan, whose ranges are based on 'musk', in fact use synthetic derivatives to keep prices down.

According to Dr Michael Green of the Conservation Monitoring Centre of the International Union for Conservation of Nature and Natural Resources in Cambridge, who studied musk deer for the World Wildlife Fund, perfumes which still contain the real thing include Chanel's *No 5*, Guerlain's *L'Heure Bleue*, Rochas' *Madam Rochas* and Shiseido's *Suzoro*. None of these actually advertise the fact, because it is not considered a redhot selling point. Indeed, when the BBC made a documentary about the musk deer in 1986, Guerlain's present head of the family apparently cancelled an interview, which was due to be included in the programme, because he decided he did not want to be associated with the trade.

The musk deer is protected to some extent by the international legislation which covers other endangered species. However, the World Wildlife Fund has found evidence that vast quantities are exported from China to Japan via Hong Kong. In 1986 alone, more than 37,000 of these endangered animals are thought to have been slaughtered to provide the 367 kilos of musk imported by Japan. More than 80 per cent of this traffic was reckoned to be contraband.

Japan is by far the biggest user of musk in the world, accounting for perhaps 85 per cent of the trade, with France buying the remainder — about 50 kilograms a year, or 500 deers' worth. No-one knows just how rare the musk deer is becoming in the world, but it is estimated that each year up to half the population is slaughtered to meet demand.

Ironically, it is possible to obtain the musk from the animals without killing them and, although the animal liberation movement may also hate the idea of 'farmed' musk, at least harvesting the musk from captive animals is preferable to their widepread illegal decimation in the wild. Unfortunately 'farming' musk is tricky because the males secrete very little when captured, especially when they are caged, as they have to be to prevent them fighting one another.

The alternative is a worldwide ban on musk, but that seems pretty unlikely in view of commercial pressures.

THE CIVET CAT

The civet cat produces civet which, like musk, is scraped from its sex glands, and this, too, is a valuable fixative for the industry. In its natural state the civet perfume is obnoxious but long-lasting, and it is only with extreme dilution that it becomes attractive.

The civet cat, like the musk deer, can be kept in captivity and the substance extracted without it having to die. Although the civet is found in large parts of India, it is the African civet which is believed to produce the best civet perfume in commercial use. Because of the recent famine in Ethiopia — one of the best natural habitats for the civet cat — worldwide stocks have been in short supply for some time now.

WHALES

The endangered sperm whale is a major source of raw materials for cosmetics in two ways. Ambergris, which is taken from the stomach of the whale, is used in many products as a fixative to help scent to last.

The substance is, in fact, coughed up by whales and can be collected from the surface of the sea. Unfortunately, despite an international campaign to save them from the bounty hunters, whales are still being slaughtered because of their valuable stomach contents, but if world opinion changed and really did want to 'Save the Whale', the cosmetics and perfume industry could still have its ambergris and the whales could still survive.

Whales also produce a wax, found in their blubber, which is used as a lubricant for lipstick and creams of all kinds.

Because the species was under threat, international moves were made to try and protect the whales, and in January 1986 a moratorium on killing whales was introduced throughout the world.

WASTE PRODUCTS

In the summer of 1987 the International Whaling Commission meeting in London was told that the major whaling nations (Iceland, South Korea, Norway, and Japan) were all exploiting a loophole in the moratorium by continuing to slaughter whales, in pursuit of 'scientific research'. Japan, the world's largest whaling nation, declared that it intended to take 1,600 minke whales and 100 sperm whales from the sea during the next two years. The Japanese prize whales more for their meat, which apparently tastes like veal, than for cosmetics, but since the whales are killed anyway, the 'waste products' are very useful for the country's extremely profitable and powerful cosmetics industry.

Scientists from the non-whaling nations insist that there is nothing we need to learn about whales which cannot be discovered without slaughtering them and that the 'research' label is merely a pretence. The World Wildlife Fund says that even if all whaling ended immediately, it could be at least 200 years before stocks of the different species are sufficiently replenished for them to be caught once more without the prospect of extinction.

There is also a lively trade in the 'waste products' of some animals, particularly in the competitive skin care industry. The cells of placenta or afterbirth taken from ewes, mares and cows have all been used in expensive skin creams, especially some of those claiming anti-ageing activities.

La Prairie, for example, a Swiss based company, uses lamb's cells in its exclusive range of skin creams, according to its saleswoman in Harrods. The cells are extracted from the placenta (afterbirth) of specially-bred black sheep, an expensive process apparently as an 'emergency treatment' of ampoules costs £129, according to La Prairie's PR, Vivienne Tomei. The Harrods consultant insisted that the live cells could delay the ageing process for about 10 years.

HUMAN INGREDIENTS?

Some people find the use of animals in cosmetics repugnant, but for others the fact that *human* parts might be contained in the pots and jars on their dressing tables is even more disgusting.

However, human placenta has, for some time, been used by the pharmaceutical industry for medical research. As it is a rich source of otherwise discarded material, few people could feel squeamish if the cosmetics industry followed suit, especially if it meant liberating a few laboratory animals from some nasty tests. A report published in the *Guardian* in 1987 noted that a French drug company was buying human placentas from 400 British maternity hospitals at a cost of 25 pence each. The average city maternity hospital makes a few hundred pounds a year from these sales. Vital tissues are extracted and used in the formulation of certain drugs which are not actually sold in Britain.

But, perhaps more gruesome than this practice is one which is the subject of regular reports — that the cosmetics industry uses human foetuses for cosmetic research. The foetuses, which are the results of abortions, are said mainly to come from France, although there are suggestions that the original sources are in the Third World. A report published by a group of European MPs in 1983 said.

> The use made of live and dead human foetuses has assumed such proportions that this phenomenon must be examined, bearing in mind the clandestine nature of such practices.

The supply of foetuses from abortions carried out in Britain is controlled by the Human Tissue Act which protects all foetuses more than 28 weeks old. Younger foetuses are used in medical research but there is no evidence that any of them find their way into cosmetics laboratories.

However, in 1985, the BBC programme *Tomorrow's World* alleged that two British companies were offering to supply non-British aborted foetuses for use in research, which included research carried out by cosmetics companies. One firm quotes a price of £40 for thymus, £102 for pituitary glands and £79 a kilogram for spleen.

Whether these reports have much foundation and, if so, how much trade there is in human parts is not known. It is certainly something that the industry would want to keep exceedingly quiet about. For obvious reasons, you would never be able to find out if any product you use has been formulated or tested in this way.

CHAPTER SEVEN

SKIN CARE

Having good skin is largely a matter of luck, as is being tall, or handsome. Some people are just born with a lovely 'peaches and cream' complexion whilst others, no matter how much money and care they lavish on their skins, still end up looking tired and prematurely wrinkly.

Cosmetics clearly have a part to play in skin care, but a smaller one than the beauty business would have us believe. A good diet, with lots of nutritious fresh food, low carbohydrates and alcohol, no smoking and lots of fresh water, all do far more good for the skin than anything you can buy in a pot.

DO YOU NEED A MOISTURIZER?

In a perfect world, with a healthy diet and lots of fresh air, without too much sun or wind there would be no need for moisturizers. But, in an imperfect polluted world, where we combine exposure to wind and strong sunshine with shutting ourselves up inside over-dry centrally-heated, air-conditioned, stuffy buildings, most of us find our skins getting dry, flakey and uncomfortably tight.

Repeated exposure to water and detergent also dries the skin, so regular bathing to wash away everyday grime also

> Only two moisturizing agents improve dry skins: sheep fat (lanolin) and petroleum jelly (vaseline).

strips the body of its natural oils. (Incidentally, your skin *should* feel tight after washing with water, according to the late Dr Erno Lazlo, who based his up-market range of skincare products on the elementary principle of washing with soap and water.)

During childhood and adolescence, few skins get dry — on the contrary, puberty and the various hormonal changes which occur can make the skin excessively oily. However, once the body has settled down, many people find their skin begins to dry up, especially by the time they reach their thirties when the skin's metabolism slows down and it becomes thinner. Even then, despite what the cosmetics industry tries to tell us, the main cause of the damage is the ageing effect of sunlight, not a deficiency in our own metabolisms. If you don't believe me, just compare the skin on parts of your body rarely or never exposed to sunlight with that on the back of your hands — however old you are!

TWO EFFECTIVE MOISTURIZING AGENTS

Skin care is controversial, but most scientists agree that only two moisturizing agents unequivocally bring about long-term improvement to dry skin — lanolin, or sheep fat, and petroleum jelly, better known as Vaseline. Both are cheap, but in their raw state these ingredients are pretty unappealing and some dermatologists reckon that Vaseline stops the skin breathing and inflames the sweat glands.

Simple *Vaseline Intensive Care* cream is both cheap and effective. It contains glycerine, petrolatum and zinc oxide — the latter colours the skin but does not penetrate it. Glycerine acts as a humectant, and although it used to be heavy and sticky, newer cosmetic formulations are lighter and easier to use. Avon's *Night Support* cream and Pond's *Cream and Cocoa Butter Lotion* both contain glycerine, for example.

A good moisturizer should contain effective protective oils, a hydrating agent or humectant, a sunscreen and above all, be suitable for your own particular type of skin. A dry skin can take a greasy formula whereas an oily skin will need an oil-free moisturizer — if it needs one at all, being naturally well-lubricated.

However, *beware*! A cream containing a humectant will only retain moisture in the skin if the outside air is damp. If it is dry, the humectant works in the opposite way and draws the moisture *out*.

Humectants usually have complicated sounding names, like propylene glycol, (which can cause allergic or toxic reactions in some people), polyethene glycol, glycerol or cholesterol.

A recent development has been the discovery that a polymer called polyglyceryl methacrylate acts as a humectant/moisture barrier and seems more effective than all the collagen, elastin and plant extracts generally found in more expensive creams.

Some people try to prevent their skin drying out either by spraying their face with a 'spritzer' from time to time, which is also very refreshing in hot weather, or by placing bowls of water around a centrally heated room or using a humidifier to stop the air drying out.

Most creams, as well as humectants, contain preservatives to prevent bacteria forming each time you dip your fingers into the pot for another 'blob'. The use of tubes minimizes the risk of contamination in this way. Some companies, which do not use preservatives, point out to their customers that the shelf life of their products is limited and stocks should be used up quickly.

Unfortunately, as British cosmetics do not have to list their ingredients, you can rarely discover what a particular skincream actually contains. The 'secret recipe' element is the basis on which they are usually sold to the customer.

Generally, the more expensive the cream, the more ingredients it contains, but this in itself may not be a good thing and indeed is more likely to cause allergic reactions than simple products. *Oil of Ulay*, for example, is a more complicated formula, containing nearly twenty different ingredients and because of this, costs around eight times as much as the *Vaseline Intensive Care* cream.

VALUE FOR MONEY

Prices for moisturizers range from about 50 pence an ounce to £50 or £60 an ounce. Most dermatologists insist that there is little difference in effectiveness between them — indeed, most recommend the cheaper creams rather than the more expensive ones.

NIGHTCREAMS

Nightcreams are usually sold with claims of being richer, and even 'nutritional', and are oilier than day creams. They are designed to be left on the skin for several hours, during a time when most people don't mind having an oily face.

Be very sceptical about claims that they 'feed' the skin, especially as *Harry's Cosmeticology*, the textbook 'bible' of the industry, is uncharacteristically dismissive of such creams:

The benefits to be expected from the

use of night creams have undoubtedly been overstated in the past. There is no doubt that the occlusive layer they provide for the skin surface slows the rate of trans-epidermal water loss and can therefore claim to have a 'moisturizing' effect...

...From time to time however, formulators have been tempted to add the term 'nutritive' to their description of such products: this is a term which can hardly be justified, irrespective of the constituents of such creams, since the *Stratum Corneum* is completely dead and any materials (such as hormones) which penetrated this layer, would, by current definition, alter the status of such a product from cosmetic to pharmaceutical.

Harry's Cosmeticology also warns:

While it is true is that many such products have been a commercial success, few have stood the test of careful scientific investigation. Preeminent among these, are 'natural' products — particularly vitamins.

The authors are sceptical about the alleged benefits of various vitamins. Quoting a lengthy list of research papers, they suggest that, on the whole, if these are to do the skin any good at all, they should be swallowed, rather than plastered on the surface where penetration is dubious and anyway of questionable benefit.

The best that can be said of vitamin E, which many people swear by, is that it might help retain some intrinsic goodness already the skin — not add anything to it.

These days, one good development is that many moisturizers contain a sunblock, often without declaring it, and since dermatologists universally agree that the sun is the single most damaging hazard to skin, it is worth searching for a moisturizer that contains a UV filter. Sometimes this is mentioned on the label but not always. The box lists some moisturizers containing UV filters.

As the only proven way to slow up the skin's ageing process is by using a sunblock and staying out of the sun (see Chapter 8), it is a bizarre feature of the industry that some companies are so coy about telling you that their moisturizers contain this useful ingredient.

HINT

Look for a moisturizer that contains a UV filter. This will help protect against harmful sunlight and premature ageing of the skin. Two examples are Guerlain's *Evolution* and Lancome's *Niosome*.

ADVICE FROM AN EXPERT

Professor Albert Kligman, a remarkably youthful-looking 70-year-old dermatologist, is one of the world's leading experts on ageing and how to combat its unattractive visible effects on the skin. He is regarded as one of the leading experts on skin care currently alive and has been Professor of Dermatology at the University of Pennsylvania for more than 30 years. I talked with him and pass on his thoughts on the skin and the cosmetics products you can buy for it so you can make up your own mind about skin care.

His basic recomendation to people of all skin types, but especially the pale Celtic ones whose complexions are apparently the most vulnerable of all, is to use two products only — petroleum jelly (or Vaseline), and a good sunblock.

A blob of Vaseline rubbed into the skin every 24 hours, together with a sunblock to protect it from the harmful effects of sunlight, are all people need to keep their skins in perfect health. In addition, they can apply anything they want to on top, including foundation and face powders — they will not harm it at all, he says.

The Professor neither rubbishes the cosmetics industry nor dismisses the concerns most people feel about the physical disadvantages of ageing skin. 'It is as foolish to dismiss all moisturizers as useless as it is to say that many of them can work miracles.'

> 'Use two products only: petroleum jelly and a good sunblock.'
> *Professor Albert Kligman*

He gets cross with medical colleagues who feel that concern over ageing skin is trivial and should not be pandered to. 'People who look prematurely aged don't feel good, they get depressed and they get sick and they need the help that some cosmetics can give them,' he says.

He points out that just as medical science has now succeeded in making us all — especially women — live longer, so it has also produced some simple key ideas on how to combat ageing skin.

One of the first things the Professor did at the university was to establish the Ivy Research Laboratory where all the major beauty companies take their new products for analysis and expert assessment by him.

Most of the products available to the public are, in his opinion, either ineffective, inappropriate or even downright dangerous. Included in these are the ones that often produce the most dramatic physical 'improvements' in the shortest possible time.

'Anything that gives such an effect within a couple of weeks or so must be causing sub-clinical injuries, which could only be visible by doing a biopsy on the skin,' he believes.

However, Professor Kligman recently lent his weighty name to endorse a new ingredient — liposomes, which became available in two up-market skin-creams in 1986. Many other experts disagree with him about liposomes.

The first of these creams was Lan-

> Most of the products available to the public are either ineffective, inappropriate or dangerous.
>
> *Professor Albert Kligman*

côme's *Niosome*, which had been developed over 14 years and which Professor Kligman said was as effective, although much nicer to use, than his beloved Vaseline. The second was Christian Dior's *Capture*.

BUYING SKIN CREAMS

The skin cream market is one of the most lucrative of all, worth an estimated £40 million a year in Britain alone. And the sector is growing more rapidly than most of the others.

We choose our face creams according to image, smell, price, mood, and above all, in a response to the hard sell. A recent study of European women showed that 70 per cent regularly use a day cream or moisturizer, while only 30 per cent use a night cream.

Another study recently showed that it was only the increasing sales of moisturizers in particular which had prevented the overall cosmetics market from levelling out in the early 1980s.

Indeed, the market might well have

slumped, as a result of increasing prices, had it not been for the heightened awareness of health and fitness which was probably the inspiration behind the demand for skin care products.

Beware of the sales assistants with their instant skin analyses! The day before I met Professor Kligman, I was accosted by a white-coated sales-assistant at one of the specialist counters in Selfridges. She asked if I wanted a skin analysis. Instead of making my usual dash for escape from any sales-person, I agreed.

She proceeded to prod my cheek a couple of times, asked if I felt my skin was 'sensitive', to which I replied 'yes', and she then started writing down a list of recommended products. At the end of the three-minute 'diagnosis', she handed me the list, which, had I bought all of the products, would have cost me over £100. But that was just the beginning, as I was to return in four or five weeks' time for a new set of products because my 'sensitive' skin would then be 'corrected' and the original products would be redundant.

When I asked Professor Kligman about this kind of approach to skin analysis, he laughed. 'It's pure hype, theatre and nonsense,' he said, adding that he had recently done a similar thing and had wandered up to a cosmetic sales assistant in Bloomingdales and asked if she could help him look 30 years younger in a 'desperate bid to win the affection of a younger woman.' (Professor Kligman, it should be added, is very happily married.)

'It was wonderful, farcical, fantastic theatre,' he said, and added that, rather than humiliate the assistant by revealing his identity, he obediently bought $200 worth of her products and promised her he would set off on his 'mission'.

His advice to the rest of us is not to be so stupid. No skin can be analysed in such a superficial way. The best advice to anyone who genuinely thinks they suffer from a sensitive skin is to stop using all the things they have been using and see if there is some *real* improvement in a month's time.

Five years ago, Professor Kligman set up The Ageing Skin Clinic. (It takes six months before you can get an appointment, which says something about the popularity of the clinic.)

SENSITIVE SKINS

Anyone who thinks she suffers from a sensitive skin should stop using any skin care products for a month.

Professor Kligman undertakes a skin analysis by slicing a sample top layer off the skin of the arm with a razor. It sounds horrible, but is quite painless because the top layer of the skin has no nerve endings in it which can register pain. He then examines the skin under a microscope and pronounces treatment. For anyone whose skin is beyond repair, he will recommend a small amount of surgical 'tidying up' — nothing too major. But his main concern is with the younger and middle-aged women (and men) who can, with the right information, protect their skins to some extent against the ravages of time. And this information is, basically, to use Vaseline and sun block.

Moisturizers, incidentally, cannot 'restructure' the skin, as is commonly claimed in the scientific blurb that accompanies the most expensive products. Nor rejuvenate an old, ugly face and make it beautiful. They merely help to prevent it drying out.

BEAUTY EDITORS DON'T HELP MUCH EITHER...

If the shop assistants don't offer us much help, nor do any of the beauty 'experts' in women's magazines. The vast majority of them just churn out re-writes of the industry's sophisticated glossy public-relations literature, without challenging it, because their expertise is literary and stylistic rather than scientific or medical.

Magazines are also provided, as I have explained, with superb colour and black and white photographs by cosmetic companies. This saves them a fortune in commissioning their own independent illustrations or editorial copy. More importantly, these magazines rely heavily on the advertising provided by cosmetic companies (see Chapter 3). The glossier the magazine, the greater the predominance of skin care ads, and, if you look carefully, you will see that their beauty write-ups tend to be the least critical. When I tried to interest some of these magazines in doing some serious consumer research, the journalists backed off at the very sound of the title of this book for fear of upsetting their advertisers.

SO WHO CAN HELP AND ADVISE ON MOISTURIZERS AND SKIN CARE?

Dermatologists are not only inaccessible, but also of little use to the average cosmetics buyer because they are trained to deal with problem skins, not ordinary skins.

The vast majority of people with ordinary skin problems have been left to the mercy of the cosmetics industry, which has the competition and its profits uppermost in its mind.

SOME TIPS ON BUYING WISELY

For a start, regard with scepticism all the products sold on the basis of hype about collagen, 'free radicals' and other pseudo-scientific terms. There is, according to dermatologists, no serious scientific evidence to support or justify these claims for products which are normally very expensive indeed. Collagen applied on the surface of the skin does not penetrate to any depth where it can actually replenish lost elasticity, despite what the skin care companies claim. All the collagen does in such creams is help the skin retain moisture, provided the atmosphere is not too dry — otherwise it loses it!

Injected collagen can supplement the natural supply and plump out the skin again. However, 'top-ups' are required every year at least.

One of the 'latest, most revolutionary' skin products is Guerlain's *Evolution* range (which claims to penetrate the layers of the skin so deeply that it can repair the DNA.). Appealing though such claims are, when I put them to Professor Kligman, he was unimpressed about the alleged 'magic' of the key ingredient Revitenol. Although he had not tried the products out himself, the data he has seen is, he says 'very seriously flawed' and the claims that Revitenol can repair damaged skin deep down are not 'scientifically verifiable'. The company naturally stands by its own research. The problem for us, the consumers, is that it is very easy for the industry to produce stunning 'before' and 'after' photographs, showing how lines and wrinkles can be removed by their products, but without a microscope and a degree in dermatology it is impossible to know whether this superficial improvement has been achieved, at the expense of causing deep-down damage, as if often the case.

After all, if you inject a prune with water you can make it look plump and young again, and so it will remain until the water dries out and it shrivels up once more.

'Cellular repair' or 'night recovery' products are on sale in other countries, especially America, and, for the time being at least, you should err on the side of scepticism rather than laying out vast sums for products whose glorious claims have failed to convince the world's independent experts. After all, if these creams really worked, wouldn't doctors be prescribing or suggesting them? Before you panic and throw away all your jars of face cream, it should be added that occasional and sparing use of these products will not harm you; it is the routine, repeated use over years and decades which the industry and sales assistants urge, which may cause permanent damage.

Unfortunately, the face needs more

> 'Nobody dies of old skin.'
>
> *Professor Kligman*

treatment than any other part of the human body. Its exposure is far greater, and its tissues more sensitive than other relatively exposed parts like the hands, feet, arms and legs. Moreover, it has to last us for a lifetime. In the past, when women rarely lived beyond the child-bearing years, it did not matter how wrinkled or dry their skin became by that time. Now our skin has to last us maybe 80 years or more and, is given much tougher treatment by the harsh unnatural environment we have created for it.

All other mammals exposed to the environment are better protected against it than we are. Our pets can lie in the sun longer than we can without it harming them, yet instinctively they move into the shade!

But, to end on a more positive note, as Professor Kligman points out, 'Nobody dies of old skin. We don't gently leak away into the environment.'

FACIALS

The function of a facial is to remove the dead cells on the surface of the skin on the face. In the old days, women used to use pumice paste and sea sand, which was a little harsh, but did much the same thing as the plethora of face-masks, grainy creams, oatmeal scrubs and even ground-up apricot shells you can now buy to carry out a facial.

One of the most effective types of facial is one you can do yourself at home, at the minimum of cost. Using a mild exfoliating cream, or just a plain old cleanser, give your face a really vigorous scrub — really massage the cleaner into all the corners, around the nose and chin — for as long as you can until you get bored, say five minutes. Then jump into a hot steamy bath and soak for up to 20 minutes. Your face will look horrible afterwards — red, puffy and decidely un-sexy, but, underneath, the skin will be really working hard to make new cells. Don't do this too often, (more frequently in winter, if your skin is dry and flakey from too much central heating and not enough fresh air).

You can also buy home facial sauna equipment for under £20, and if your skin is bad, this might be a good investment. The equipment is also useful for clearing stuffy heads in winter when your nasal tubes are blocked and uncomfortable. A bit of eucalyptus oil in the tray cleanses the tubes and the skin on the face at the same time. Just the thing for a cold wet evening when there's nothing on the TV and your skin is looking so grim that even make-up can't work as a temporary disguise! But a jug of steaming hot water and a towel over your head works just as well.

A professional facial will usually last anything up to an hour and cost up to £20. Just as a visit to the hairdresser can be relaxing and therapeutic, so too can a visit to a beautician for a facial. A professional will always massage the face after cleansing and this will leave the skin feeling good and get the circulation going. Good cosmetics companies often offer 'free' facials providing you buy a stipulated minimum of their products afterwards.

Just as you can rarely, if ever, find out what products the hairdresser uses on your hair, nor can you find out what the professional beautician uses in her routine, although she may tell you some of the ingredients. Many use a paraffin-based mask, which sounds revolting and is not recommended for home use. This sets into a kind of skin of its own and pulls off the dead cells when it is removed.

The skin will then be very dry and will be moisturized and even 'fed' with a 'nourishing' cream. It may not do all that the beautician claims it will do, but your skin will be feeling so tight that some sort of moisturizer is necessary.

CLEANSERS VERSUS SOAP AND WATER

The cosmetics industry and the dermatologists will never agree on whether it is better to use good old fashioned soap and water to scrub the face clean or instead to buy one of the many cleansers now available for all skin types.

Because so many cleansers contain fragrance and other ingredients which can make the skin itch and feel irritated, the simplest and cheapest solution for most people is to use an unperfumed soap with water and to resort to cleansers only if your face feels taut and uncomfortable for more than an hour or so afterwards.

Dermatologists reckon soap and warm water is the best way of cleaning the skin. However, cleansers can be handy if you are travelling and want to remove the grime and freshen up without the convenience of a wash-basin and clean towels. If you wear make-up, soap and water won't always remove it — particularly if it contains grease.

Some manufacturers now make non-soap 'soaps' or complexion bars which are quite effective in cleansing the face. They are solid versions of cleansing creams rather than traditional soap and much less harsh. These 'soaps', do not condition or moisturize the skin. Antiseptic soaps have little lasting effect as any drying or anti-bacterial agent is lost once the product is washed off the face.

Unfortunately, when the skin is cleaned with any strong substance, the natural protective oils are stripped along with the grease and grime. Most human skin has a pH level of between 4.5 and 5.5, which makes it slightly acidic. As anyone who vaguely remembers their chemistry lessons will know, alkaline substances can break down acids and therefore if cosmetics which contains alkaline ingredients are constantly being used, the skin's natural pH balance can be destroyed. This can lead to dehydration, the production of fine lines or wrinkles, irritation and a reduced resistence to spots and other infections. Dermatologist Dr Patricia Engasser of the University of California says that as cleansers remove oils which protect the skin, using cleansers regularly leaves the skin prone to problems such as dryness, irritation, contact dermatitis and acne. Dr Marianne O'Donoghue, Associate Professor of Dermatology at Rush Presbyterian St Luke's Medical Center in Chicago insists that soap and water are the best cleansing agents. 'I advise all my patients to use a mild soap rinsed off with water, and I tell them not to use a moisturizer unless they have to,' she told a skin care conference in London in 1988.

All of this means that if you do use a cleanser to remove dirt, you should afterwards use a skin tonic or freshener to remove that. Skin products tend to be sold in sets because you can't use one without the others! (Rather like hair products, once you start dyeing and perming, you have to use conditioners . . .)

Some people find that a combination works best for them and they can use an oily-based cleanser to get rid of oil-based make-up, and then freshen up with a splash of soap and water. If you don't use oily make-up and your skin is either dry or normal, then soap and water should be quite sufficient, followed by a moisturizer if you feel you need to use one.

WHICH CLEANSER FOR YOU?

For those who need or prefer to use cleansers, oily skins are best cleaned with a milky cleansing lotion which removes the dirt without adding grease, while dry skins sometimes need an oilier substance to remove dirt without taking precious moisture with it. A pharmacist, rather than sales assistant, should be able to advise on this, otherwise you can experiment by using trial sizes. Tubes are the most hygenic containers, incidentally, as anything like a jar which you dip your fingers in becomes contaminated the minute you start to use it.

Incidentally, whatever cleanser you buy, the major ingredient will be water. Other ingredients usually include beeswax, mineral oil and borax. There is no evidence that the more expensive cleansers are any better than the cheaper ones, so an economy tube or jar or chain store 'own brand' is probably fine for most people. Unless you absolutely cake yourself in make-up, it should last for months. If you use oil-based eye make-up then a water-based cleanser or soap and water may not make much impression. Waterproof mascaras — if they are doing their job — should be impossible to shift without oil. Oily pads are a convenient method, but these contain more oil than you would choose yourself and can be messy.

A reasonably oily cleansing cream like Ponds should suffice. If you wear contact lenses, take them out first before using an oily make-up remover or the results can be painful. Getting oil off lenses is no easy task either.

Having said this, I rarely bother to use a special eye make-up remover and have always found that whatever I use on the rest of my face usually cleans the areas around the eyes too, but then I don't wear heavy-duty make up.

ASTRINGENTS

Astringents are variously described as 'toners', 'pore closers', or something similarly scientific. In fact, all they are

> Witch hazel is a natural astringent. A year's supply costs about £1. Buy it from a chemist.

is alcohol mixed perhaps with witch hazel. Witch hazel is a natural astringent and if such a compound is needed at all, a large bottle from the chemist should be enough to supply most people for a year or more and costs less than a pound. Similarly, many so-called 'toners' are 50 per cent water and almost as much again rose water, which can also be bought from the chemist for a few pence.

Astringents are designed and sold to eliminate the oiliness which is usually only present on the face as a direct result of using other types of cosmetics — specifically moisturizers and night-creams, but also oil-based cleansers.

Products containing too much alcohol can be *too* drying and irritate the skin. Only people with very oily skins find them useful.

The cosmetics industry's claims that astringents 'tighten the skin' and 'close the pores' are misleading. They can only have a temporary and therefore an inconsequential effect.

EXFOLIATORS

Dermatologists disagree about the usefulness of exfoliation, that is, getting rid of the surface dead cells. On the one hand, some say that buffing the skin can stimulate new growth of cells, temporarily plump it up and make superficial wrinkles less obvious. It can also help loosen and remove blackheads and keep pores unblocked so other spots do not form.

On the other hand, some say that exfoliation can be too rough for sensitive or dry skin and, if done too vigorously, it can worsen skin problems like acne. Dr John Harper, a dermatologist at Great Ormond Street Hospital says of exfoliators: 'These products are potent irritants and most people who use them experience some irritation.'

What is also true is that no moisturizer will be able to do its job — however good the product — if the skin is not receptive to treatment. A dull greyish complexion may be a sign that dead cells are clinging to the surface, making it difficult for creams to penetrate and do even the most superficial of maintenance jobs. It takes up to a month for the top layer of skin to shed itself completely.

The cosmetics market is brimming with various exfoliation products, from grainy substances like ground-up walnut shells (which are too harsh for sensitive skins) to gentle herbal 'peeling' creams which, with a flannel, help remove dead cells from sensitive skins.

The only way you can find out if exfoliation is going to help your own skin is by trial and error. If afterwards your skin feels taut or irritated, then you are being too tough on it. For most people exfoliation can be carried out without any commercial products, simply by using a flannel or a sponge — and the oilier their skin, the more often they should do it. However, flannels and sponges should be regularly washed or boiled to

> 'I'm a big advocate of using a
> wash-cloth... I do think it
> removes a lot of grit and
> bacteria'
> *Dr John Romano*

keep them scrupulously clean because, if you are shifting deeply-embedded dirt in one wash, you don't want to re-apply it in the next.

'I'm a big advocate of using a wash-cloth — there's just some material you're not going to get off by casual washing with your hands,' says Dr John Romano, dermatologist at the New York Hospital Cornell Medical Center. 'I do think it removes a lot of grit and bacteria, so you don't develop the little whiteheads that are definitely related to debris on the face'.

Incidentally, suntanning causes exfoliation, because the flaking tan is a megadose of the process. However, as we shall see, it is also very ageing.

CHAPTER EIGHT

ANTI-AGEING 'WONDERCREAMS'

There has been a spate of new 'anti-ageing' creams launched on the cosmetics market in the last couple of years, with phials of this and potions of that, bits of mare's placenta, extracts of cells of newborn lambs and so on, each of whose inventor has claimed to have 'at last' found the secret ingredient of everlasting youth.

The cosmetics companies have all realized that women have suddenly become aware of the damage they have been doing to their faces by all those years of suntanning, and that ordinary moisturizers don't seem to be having any effect on all those fine wrinkles (How can they?).

Most experts will agree with dermatologists like Dr Tina Green of Addenbrookes Hospital, Cambridge, who says, 'The problem is that we cannot make older skin look like younger skin.'

However, the cosmetics companies want us to believe otherwise — that buffing and exfoliating and regenerating cells with all sorts of ingredients can somehow restore a baby-skinned complexion. They vie with each other in producing scientific 'data' to support their particular anti-ageing 'secrets'.

THE 'SCIENTIFIC DATA' GAME

To do this, they employ laboratories to formulate the products and test them, hence the claims 'scientifically formulated', 'dermatologically tested', etc.

> 'We cannot make older skin look like younger skin'
> *Dr Tina Green*

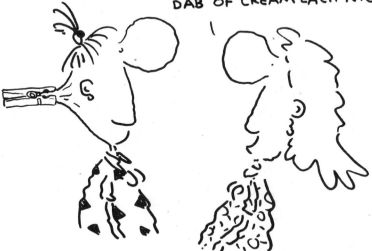

SURELY THERE'S MORE TO IT THAN JUST A LITTLE DAB OF CREAM EACH NIGHT.

What the cosmetics companies and their public relations teams choose to do with such results is their own affair, and it appears that the slightest positive word from the laboratories sends them into ecstasies of prose which refer, though not specifically, to their 'scientific data'. It is very hard to obtain copies of this data to assess it, so one has to rely on their honesty and interpretation of the results.

In such a competitive world it is hardly uncharitable to suggest that the claims made are out of all proportion to the results found. The fact that these companies keep coming out with *new* anti-ageing formulas suggests that they themselves recognize that they have not yet found the magic ingredient, despite their previous claims.

La Prairie, which makes anti-ageing creams using cells from the placentas attached to newborn lambs, emphasize its Swiss laboratories in its promotional material. Thousands of patients from all over the world flock to La Prairie's clinic on the shores of Lake Geneva, for live cell transplants which they are convinced will ensure eternal youth. Lesser mortals can pay £129 for a 28-day rejuvenation course which they can use in their own bathrooms.

To buy a full range of La Prairie skin care products would cost literally hundreds of pounds, but those who cannot afford it should not feel too left out. Although nobody has done the research, a jar of any old cream may do you just as much good, if you believe it will.

THE 'IS IT A DRUG, THEN?' DILEMMA

Cosmetic companies find themselves in something of a dilemma, for if their products really *can* drastically alter the nature of skin cells, as they often suggest they can, then they are, technically speaking, dealing with a drug, which should be subject to all sorts of independent tests so that such claims can be substantial by the experts — in this case the dermatologists.

If they do not want to go down this road, and none do, then they have to fudge the wording so that they can still claim the products are cosmetics, that is, skin deep, rather than drugs, which are more powerful.

Anti-ageing creams, if they are to work, must reach down below the epidermis of the skin, which accounts for the top 10 per cent, to the dermis, where collagen and elastin and the support system operates, and where the signs of ageing begin. But, since this is the layer where the skin protects itself from outside invaders, interfering with it is be potentially dangerous, according to some dermatologists.

As mentioned in the last chapter, 'liposomes' were the headline skin story of 1986, with both Lancôme and Christian Dior producing anti-ageing creams containing these 'magic' ingredients which, if the 'scientific' claims are to be believed, work deep down in the epidermis, stimulating new cells to regenerate.

When they were launched, they provoked immediate criticism from dermatologists outside the industry, including Dr Green, who said, 'It perplexes me that cosmetics companies are spending so much time and money on liposomes because, to incorporate the inter-cellular components liposomes carry, cells have to be able to take on board outside molecules, and most skins cannot do this.'

Mine, incidentally, must be one of the unlucky ones, because in over a year of using Lancôme's *Niosome*, I can detect no improvement. However, when I mentioned this to a Lancôme sales assistant in Harrods, whilst obtaining a trial sample and blurb about their very latest new product *Oligo-Major*, I was assured the results were long term and that I would not expect to see any noticeable difference yet. It is very hard to argue with that. Perhaps the fact that I can't see any difference means that they have achieved their object — in other words, my skin has not got any older-looking in a year!

Lancôme's new product comes in a medicinal-looking brown bottle and acts as a 'cellular bio-activating serum' which is said to stimulate the skin into extra activity, so much so 'that you can feel your skin responding from the very first application'. Mine responds more to a splash of cold water.

Charles of the Ritz produces an anti-ageing product, called *Age-Zone Controller*, which is said to produce a 34 per cent reduction in wrinkles. However, this is only an average figure and Dr John Seibert of Charles of the Ritz admits, 'It will reduce some people's lines by maybe five per cent; others by maybe 80 per cent.' Again, I could discern no difference using my trial sample but I daresay that again, this is something the company would insist one had to use for some length of time.

Estée Lauder, with its *Prescriptives* range, claim to take the liposome action even further than Lancôme or Dior, by improving the delivery system which had been so heavily criticized by dermatologists.

Meanwhile, dermatologists hired by Helena Rubinstein to launch their brand-new anti-ageing range *Perfor-mance* H_2O are confusing everyone still more by claiming that the level of greasiness in the skin has nothing to do with the amount of water it contains or retains, thus rejecting all the previous rules about the three skin types, oily, normal and dry. Overturning several established beliefs about human skin, they say that the amount of moisture in the skin is determined by the amount in the atmosphere, with extremes of cold and heat, the drying effects of central heating and air conditioning being important determining factors.

They also insist that the skin does *not* get drier with age. Dry skin is something we are genetically lumbered with, and it is only altered by how we live and what we do to it.

The new Rubinstein products are therefore sold with the help of a machine which sits on the sale counter and measures the water content of potential purchasers' skins. For example, they say that a variation in temperature of 7 degrees centigrade — either way — can bring about a moisture change of 100 per cent. This product is too new for independent dermatologists to have had a chance to evaluate it.

Using the same theory, but a different approach, the Revlon scientists have been working on a new formula, designed to keep moisture in by using a layer of silicone to protect the skin from both dehydration and pollution.

ANTI-AGEING MAKE-UP?

It had to happen that the industry which had previously thought up tinted moisturizers, which added colour at the same time as moisture, has now come up with foundations which also contain 'anti-ageing' ingredients.

Revlon was one of the first companies to produce a foundation loaded with anti-ageing ingredients. No sooner was this announced than several other leading companies announced launches, or plans for launches of similar products. For example, Boots launched their *No 7 Special Collection Collagen Complex Foundation* in 1987, claiming that it did 'more than merely colour the skin . . . being a highly effective treatment product that improves skin texture while you are wearing it.'

This foundation also contains a UV filter, which is a good thing and certainly can justify the claim 'anti-ageing', as does Yardley's rival product, launched around the same time, *Satin Finish*. This also contains collagen, moisturizers and sunscreens.

If you are going to buy and wear a foundation anyway, it seems worth giving these products a try, as long as you realize they won't *remove* wrinkles. However they may help protect your skin against new ones forming quite so quickly. The box contains a list of foundations which contain a sun screen. If your favourite foundation isn't there, ask a sales assistant or the manufacturer about it.

HINT

If you wear foundation, look for one that contains a sunscreen. For example:
- *No 7 Special Collection Collagen Complex Foundation (Boots)*
- *Satin Finish (Yardley)*
- *More than Moisture (Mary Quant)*
- *Tinted Moisturizer (Colorfast)*
- *Ultra-moist make-up (Max Factor)*

DRUGS THAT COMBAT AGEING SKIN

One ingredient which might justify the description 'wonder-cream' is one that is cheap and readily available and upon which considerable research has already been done. This is retinoic acid, a synthetic derivative which is cheap to produce because it comes from vitamin A.

It is already recommended as a good treatment for severe acne, but is available in Britain on prescription only. This is because, unfortunately, it does have side-effects, in that it thins the outer layer of the skin. (Rather like the 'chemical peel' in cosmetic surgery, see page 237). Because of this, people who use retinoic acid have to protect their faces with a sunblock whenever they are in the sun, or indeed outside at all, because the face becomes very sensitive to burning.

Professor Kligman is enthusiastic about retinoic acid and he believes it not only helps to prevent ageing but can reverse its effects. Unfortunately, acid can also cause the skin to itch and redden and flake, so its use has to be limited and carefully monitored.

Needless to say, American women have been begging dermatologists to supply them with retinoic acid purely as an anti-ageing cream and some in the profession are certainly doing so. Some cosmetic scientists are already working on creams which will include retinoic acid whilst others have already included vitamin A.

The very latest research on drugs which combat ageing has been done at the University of Michigan and although the results are based on only 30 individuals, the media response has been enthusiastic.

The drug — a type of retinoic acid/ vitamin A compound called tretinoin cream, has been found, in a controlled study, to reduce the damage inflicted by the sun in the form of wrinkles, roughness and freckles.

The American Medical Association says:

> 'Researchers think the drug works by thickening the epidermis, the skin's outer layer, as well as by increasing the formation of collagen in the dermis, the layer below,'

ness and freckles. 'Researchers think the drug works by thickening the epidermis, the skin's outer layer, as well as by increasing the formation of collagen in the dermis, the layer below,' says the American Medical Association.

But before everyone rushes out to try and obtain this drug, further testing is still needed as this was an extremely limited trial conducted over only four months. At the end of the project, virtually all the patients who had used the tretinoin therapy suffered dermatitis or inflammation of the skin.

Only research over a longer period of time will show if the risks outweigh the benefits, and as this is undoubtedly a drug and not a cosmetic, it will take some time to convince the authorities. But if they do, it will be worth waiting for and you can be sure that the drug companies will package this cream as an anti-ageing formula.

GLYCEL

Of all the anti-ageing products, none was hyped more than Glycel. Launched in 1986, it was a skin cream containing a natural extract called glycosphingolipid (GSL), an ingredient which carried an impressive endorsement by Dr Christiaan Barnard, the famous heart surgeon who carried out the world's first heart transplant in 1967.

Glycel was launched with a terrific fanfare — ads in the up-market Sunday supplements — and exclusive sale in Harrods. About a year later it was quietly withdrawn from sale after a furore broke out in America over the ever more outrageous claims made for anti-ageing 'miracle creams'. Basically the authority that controls cosmetics in the US, the Food and Drug Administration, challenged the makers of products like Glycel and told them to either prove scientifically that their products worked as powerfully as they claimed or withdraw them and re-label them. In Britain, the products were simply removed from the shelves.

However, it is worth covering the Glycel story in a little detail because many people presumably have some very expensive partially-used pots in their dressing tables and are wondering why they cannot buy any more and whether they should continue to use what they have. Rest assured, the criticism of Glycel is that it was not what it claimed to be — effective in reducing wrinkles on the face, not that it was intrinsically unsafe. To some of his colleagues — and the public — Dr Barnard

lost much of his medical credibility by apparently 'selling out' to a cosmetics company. He put it quite bluntly when he admitted at the official British launch of Glycel: 'Things about me have always been very saleable.'

From 1983, severe arthritis had made it impossible for him to carry on as a surgeon, and being somewhat obsessed with the sustaining of youth, he turned his attention to skin care.

According to the PR blurb issued at the launch, which was faithfully repeated in the beauty columns of all the gullible glossy magazines, GSL was discovered in the laboratories of the Schaefer Institute in Basle, Switzerland, where cell biologists were working on various substances which might overcome the rejection problems which have beset the organ transplant programme around the world.

Dr Barnard says he found that GSL was more abundant in younger skin than older skin and it was realized instantly that this ingredient had enormous commercial potential as a 'cosmetic', so it was immediately patented. It had, in fact, been discovered by a scientist in 1874!

Unfortunately, as is usual at such product launches, the press pack had no scientific data at all and the information issued about the product merely listed the various creams available, their prices and how to use them. Glycel was turned into a cosmetic by a company called

Alfin fragrances, a small firm, hitherto specializing in perfumes and fragrances.

Its chairman, Irwin Alfin, said at the launch that despite some early side-swiping from jealous rivals and one or two 'ill-informed' dermatologists, 'business had been super.' Just how super, he explained, could be seen in the sales figures with the products yielding $12 million in America in the first three months of marketing. Mr Irwin Alfin admitted candidly: 'I don't know how GSL works. I haven't proved it.'

Denying Dr Barnard had received a rumoured sum already worth $4 million, Irwin Alfin said that the heart specialist was receiving 3.5 per cent of 5 per cent, which works out at about $135,000 for that period alone, which is not bad for a side-line. Sales were expected to top $30 million in 1986 alone, so the sums can be tripled.

On the other hand, it is perhaps not much of a price if Dr Barnard's reputation as a physician is tarnished, and the sums compare badly alongside figures like the $487,000 earned by Joan Collins for her endorsement of the fragrance *Scoundrel*, and other famous actors and actresses who endorse make up and perfume. Perhaps it would be more charitable to say that someone has got to pay for his research and this was one way of funding it.

He also refuted statements by British dermatologists who had ridiculed Glycel and suggested that it could not possibly penetrate the deeper layers of the skin because the molecules were too big.

He and Dr Barnard replied by comparing the molecules in collagen to 'the size of a grapefruit, whereas the glycel lipid is the size of a grain'. In other words, collagen doesn't work.

On the other hand, Alfin Fragrance did not prove its products worked either. Because of fears that the FDA would crack down on skin care producers who make unsupported scientific claims for their products, the company was careful to make very few specific claims for Glycel.

It did not need to.

A $2 million budget for the advertising launch together with exclusive marketing at an expensive price resulted in booming sales. On the first day it went on sale in Harrods in London more than £5,000 worth was snapped up.

Most customers were buying the 'starter's kits' at £150 each. Even Harrods' customers baulked at shelling out the £335 required for the full range of nine products.

Several statements made by Mr Alfin contradicted one another:
Compare:

'No other rival product has had as much research as ours.'

'We make almost no specific claims — this is a cosmetic not a drug.'

'No other product has ever had such attention as ours.'

'Ours is a really superior product — we can prove it.'

'Our claims are lighter and softer than almost everybody else's.'

So after all the hype and exclusivity, exactly what was the company claiming for Glycel?

Merely this: that their vastly superior product would repair the damage done to the skin by the environment. Not rejuvenate it, just nourish and texturize.

In other words, do what every other 'inferior' moisturizer claims to do!

As for the price, well at £35 a 1.7 ounce jar for the GSL Cellular Treatment Activator and £45 an ounce for the day cream and £50 an ounce for night-cream, I think it must have been the most expensive range yet. A dozen applications reduced my jar down to nearly half-way, which worked out at at least £2 a go. It sinks in pretty fast, so it's no use thinking it will last — as some creams do — for ages.

So, what could be said in Glycel's favour — compared with many rival anti-ageing formulas? Well, precious little except for one thing, and that was that the products were labelled, so you could, theoretically, find out roughly what you were putting on your face. This is rare in the mystifying world of anti-ageing potions so I thought it worth investigating with the help of a 'mole'.

For the record, the ingredients included collagen, a protein found in skin fibre which allegedly helps it retain moisture; elastin, which apparently improves skin tone; together with extracts of jasmine, mimosa, linden mallow, ginseng, jojoba and calendula. All nice natural flowery-sounding names which are certainly more appealing than a long list of chemicals.

I asked a manufacturing chemist, now retired after 21 years working in the cosmetics business, what he made of the product, and if he could copy it. Of course we do not know if the FULL ingredients were listed.

He read the list of ingredients listed on the 'Cellular Treatment Activator' and said most of them had already been widely used in other skin products, e.g. elastin and collagen. He suspected the ingredient called *proteine animale et ceramide glycoslylée* contained either extracts from human or bovine intestines or placenta, but we agreed it could have been anything, including lanolin (sheep fat), which some other dermatologists had claimed it contained when they analysed its ingredients after the launch.

Summarizing, he said that there were

so many already existing ingredients contained in the product it would be impossible to claim which was causing what effect. The only missing ingredient was of course the secret formula, GSL itself, but even if that were known, it would be impossible to make up the identical cream without having the 'recipe'.

He did stress that as the company was able to buy all the ingredients in bulk and that most of them were pretty cheap, for example, demineralized and sterilized water and glycerine, making the overall 'recipe' would not be expensive.

Okay, so Alfin Fragrances have had to pay for five years of Dr Barnard's scientific research in a Swiss laboratory and no one would pretend that comes cheap.

In the absence of any scientific data, comparing Glycel to any other product *not* containing GSL — which was not made available either to the FDA or to the public at any time — it is impossible to say whether the product is superior, or even equal to, any of the vastly cheaper alternatives.

Similarly, it is also impossible to assess whether the product could, in the long-term, even be harmful. We just don't know. But what's more significant is that, apparently, neither do they.

So, why were we all left with the impression that this was a miracle anti-ageing potion, developed in a high-powered Swiss laboratory, by top scientists working at the forefront of medical knowledge and that the whole advertising and marketing strategy combined to make this seem like the final answer to the banishment of ugly, unattractive wrinkles?

The answer of course, is because it wasn't. It was just the latest, and perhaps the most extravagant. In this case the hype went so far it stung the powerful FDA into action and forced the clampdown on such claims that cosmetics' manufacturers had been dreading. Perhaps Dr Barnard has inadvertently done us all a favour which is that in future, such products will not be able to get away with such outrageous and unscientifically verifiable claims.

Whoever invents the real thing will be not only guaranteed a fortune, but will have every dermatologist in the world leaping up and down with excitement, anxious to do trials and research on his or her own patients. Meanwhile, fortunes are being made from our gullability.

ACNE

Common acne includes blackheads, whiteheads and pimples and is caused by a chronic inflammation of the sebaceous glands, affecting primarily the face, the chest and the back.

It is the second most common widespread incurable illness (first is the common cold) and, although it has been estimated that up to 98 per cent of the population suffers from it at sometime between the age of 13 and 23, when it strikes hard its physical and psychological effects can be devastating. It is a very cruel trick of nature that acne afflicts people at a time in their lives when they are usually most self-conscious and desperate to look attractive and appealing to their friends and to the opposite sex.

Acne is popularly believed to be aggravated by certain foods and drinks — chocolate, peanuts, fizzy drinks, sweets and even cheese, all rather popular with the age group most affected. So as a precaution, anyone affected by an attack of acne should try cutting out all of these things. However, although doing this helps many people, many others don't improve, so don't get upset if such deprivation makes no odds! (There will, however, be other health benefits from cutting out these things.)

There are also a large number of products on the market designed to 'deep cleanse', 'prohibit', 'cure' and otherwise tackle acne. Advertising for this section of the market is quite extensive because the industry is aware of the numbers of people affected and the desperation of the sufferers.

Be wary of any anti-acne products which emphasize their 'antiseptic' qualities because spots are generally caused by over-active sebaceous oil glands, *not* by bacteria, so keeping your skin sterile isn't going to make any significant difference and the antiseptic lotions may cause irritation and redness and so make the problem worse rather than better.

Products which claim to help unblock the pores are more sensible and you should look for those which contain an ingredient called Recorcinol or salicylic acid. These include lotions like *Clearasil*, *DDD* and a host of other anti-spot products. Although these products may help, do not be surprised if they make no appreciable difference — some skin experts are sceptical of them, saying they do not reach the layers of the skin where spots are created anyway.

IMPORTANCE OF REGULAR WASHING

You do not necessarily need any special lotions, as regular washing of the skin with an ordinary, preferably unperfumed, soap will keep the pores unblocked and really help keep down the number of spots. So will good hygiene generally — and, whatever you do, *don't pick spots* as this only makes them worse.

If your spots are bad you should go to your doctor. Although many doctors are still rather old fashioned and tend to regard acne as something you will grow out of, he or she may prescribe either antibiotics or tetracyclines, which are effective in most cases. These are generally not prescribed too readily, especially not to girls who may become pregnant, because of potential risks to a foetus. These drugs are about 90 per cent effective, but it may take up to six months for the acne to clear completely according to a recent report in *Doctor* magazine.

Medicinal creams are also effective, especially ones containing retinoic acid, which is the acidic form of vitamin A. (Despite claims by some manufacturers, vitamin A taken in *oral* doses is not thought to make any difference to acne).

Some hormonal therapies may correct the imbalances which may trigger acne, and these include some types of the contraceptive Pill. However, few doctors will prescribe the Pill on this basis unless the affliction is especially severe and nothing else seems to work. Just to confuse matters, other types of contraceptive pill can actually *cause* spots in some unlucky women.

Lastly, the corticosteroids can also be useful, but are generally required in quite high doses to combat acne effectively. It is now possible to buy hydrocortisone creams over the counter but since these have only recently ceased to be prescription-only drugs, it is wise to consult a pharmacist before using them, and then use them sparingly maybe only once or twice a week.

Some people use sunlamps and ultraviolet radiation to help clear up acne, and although this may help, they should be aware of the other risks associated with this type of exposure. Similarly, many teenagers find that the summer sunshine and salty seawater does marvels for their spotty skins.

For those for whom nothing works, one can only offer the somewhat unsatisfactory consolation that this is something that they *will* grow out of eventually, and to try and ensure that for them the scars are only skin-deep. (Real scars, incidentally, can be removed by cosmetic surgery and if they are really disfiguring, this can be done on the NHS).

CAMOUFLAGE?

Unfortunately, tempting as it is to try to cover up one's spots, this is the worst thing anyone can do for a really bad skin. This option is not available to boys anyway, but girls should be careful as they may make their condition worse by blocking the pores. Tough as it may sound, avoiding make-up will help the spots to clear up.

What *is* helpful, in my opinion, is a good spot cover-up stick, to cover the worst offenders. Choose one which is medicated, with a drying action, so you are doing some good at the same time.

No anxious spotty teenager (male or female) should be without one, and there are several good and quite cheap ones on the market. Be sure to blend the cream carefully, and only use it sparingly during the day.

At other times, try and keep your face scrupulously clean, washing three times a day with warm water, soap and a clean soft flannel. Wash properly, don't just flick the soap and water over the skin. There is no convincing proof that specially formulated acne soap is any better than a good unperfumed soap. Many people find baby soap the best. Nor are soaps containing antibacterial agents helpful, because they do not penetrate into the skin to the levels where acne is actually caused. Do not use perfumed soaps as the amount of washing you have to do could set up an irritation and make matters worse.

Acne sufferers should wash their hair regularly (they may have to anyway because fate often combines a spotty skin with greasy hair) and they should avoid all oily hair and skin products (including suntan oils) and keep the skin as dry as possible.

Whiteheads and blackheads can be squeezed but only with scrupulously clean fingers. If it is done at night the reddening has time to fade.

Special blackhead and whitehead-removal gadgets can be bought and these are usually quite efficient at releasing the spot. Mop up afterwards with something soothing or medicated.

OTHER SKIN PROBLEMS

Unfortunately, there are many other types of skin problems, the most common being dermatitis, eczema and psoriasis. Their causes are complicated and can certainly be triggered by the action on the skin of cosmetics, soaps, shampoos, perming lotions, hair dyes, and scents. If the source of the irritation is pinpointed and then avoided, the problem will usually clear up.

Psoriasis affects about one in fifty people and those who suffer have a hyper-active skin for reasons that are not really understood. The problem can affect patches of the skin or the whole body and, like dermatitis and eczema, can be horribly itchy and unpleasant. Because the cause has not been identified, there is no cure, but avoiding all irritants, such as perfumed cosmetics and toiletries is one possible remedy.

Doctors are the best people to consult about any of these skin problems. Stay clear of the cosmetics counters as the staff will almost certainly be clueless about your condition and their products will not help you. Skin specialists may be able to do something to make the condition manageable or even make it go away if you can identify and avoid a particular substance to which you are sensitive.

CHAPTER NINE

SUNTANNING IS DANGEROUS

The sun is bad for your skin, and too much sunbathing can cause you skin cancer.

Although for centuries it was fashionable to have a pale white skin — for the past 50 or 60 years it has been quite the opposite way round and now it is widely considered desirable to sport a tan as a form of conspicuous expenditure.

Strong sunshine activates melanin in the skin which rises to the surface and gives it a tan. At the same time, the skin thickens and stretches so that, when the tan fades, the skin is more leathery and prone to fine wrinkles — the early sign of ageing.

SUNBATHING AND SKIN CANCER

Increasingly, many of us have become vaguely aware that *excess* sunbathing could damage the skin, but we all thought skin cancer was relatively harmless and, at worst, would only necessitate a brief visit to hospital as an out-patient to have a few brownish patches removed.

Wrong! Last year more than 1,000 people died in Britain from malignant melanoma, a preventable and curable form of skin cancer. Moreover, in the last 15 years, the number of such deaths has doubled as more fair-skinned people have insisted on basking in the hot sun for weeks on end and some cancer experts now believe skin cancer could become as common as breast cancer if figures continue to rise at this rate.

Women are twice as likely to develop malignant melanoma as men, and the group facing the highest risk is the middle-aged. Although twice as many women contract skin cancer as men, proportionally fewer women die — perhaps because they are more conscious of the disfigurement and go to the doctor earlier for diagnosis and treatment. On recent statistics, roughly half the women diagnosed as having malignant melanoma *die*, while two thirds of the men lose their lives.

MALIGNANT MELANOMA- THOSE MOST AT RISK

● Short sharp exposure to the sun is most dangerous, for example, intensive sunbathing on holiday for those not normally exposed to the sun.
● The middle-aged are the most vulnerable age group.
● Women are twice as likely to develop melanoma as men.
● People with fair skin, blue eyes and fair or red hair are at the greatest risk of all.

In Australia, where the highest rates of skin cancer in the world have been recorded, men and women suffer equally. An intensive public information campaign has been under way for some time, alerting fair-skinned people to the dangers of the Australian sun.

At greatest risk of all are those with fair skin and fair or red hair and blue eyes. Dark-haired, dark-skinned people rarely get skin cancer, because their skin is more resistent to the sun.

Short sharp exposure is the most dangerous. People who go in for short, intensive sunbathing sessions, on a fortnight's holiday in unfamiliarly strong sunshine for example, are at more risk of skin cancer than outdoor workers whose skin seems to build up a resistance to the sun. Latitude, altitude and the time of the day are all important factors. Skiers on high mountain slopes in thin atmospheres are in most danger, and clearly the midday sun is the strongest.

Despite the spiralling death rate, for the most part the public remains blissfully unaware of the problem, and sufferers put their lives at risk by not seeking diagnosis and treatment early on. The only good news is that, if this type of cancer is caught early, before it starts to spread into other parts of the body, there is a more than 90 per cent chance of cure, even though victims will still need to be monitored. But if the cancer, which resembles an active mole on the skin, is allowed to reach a certain thickness, the chances of surviving even the next five years plummet to 40 per cent.

SKIN CANCER STUDIES

The skin cancer problem has been studied mostly in Canada, North America, Australia and Northern Europe, where the skin cancer epidemic has been highest. It has afflicted fair-skinned caucasians who have moved about the globe, either permanently through emigration, or temporarily, on holiday to the hot sun, that is, from countries where the sun is weak and the climate is not normally conducive to sunbathing on a scale that is potentially fatal, to hot, sunny countries.

Information collected over the last twenty years shows that most skin cancer is confined to those of North European descent. In Scandinavia, skin cancer cases are doubling each decade, while in sun-baked New Mexico and Arizona, some reports suggest the incidence is quadrupling every decade. The Australian epidemic is confined almost exclusively to people who emigrated to that country from Northern Europe — most of the population.

In 1984, the *British Medical Journal* published first reports of the largest study ever carried out into skin cancer. Nearly 1,000 sufferers living in Western Canada were identified and monitored by a team of scientists and compared with similar individuals who had not developed skin cancer.

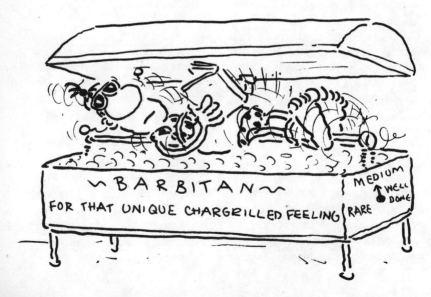

RISK FACTORS AND DANGER SIGNS

They found that light hair, skin and eye colour and a history of heavy freckling in adolescence, plus a tendency to burn readily and develop freckles and moles after sunbathing were all major risk factors. Cancer was found to develop from existing moles. Incidence was also higher among those with a family history of skin cancer.

By far the largest common factor was blonde hair — natural blondes were calculated to be seven times more vulnerable than people with dark hair. Blueness of the eyes and the paleness of unexposed skin were also found to be key indicators of risk.

So if you have naturally blonde hair, blue eyes, pale unexposed skin which freckles easily and tans poorly, resign yourself to being either naturally pale or using a fake tan if you want to appear bronzed.

In another study carried out by dermatologists in Glasgow and Edinburgh, and published in the *BMJ* in June 1986, it was found that the risk of skin cancer increased the more moles there were on a person's body. For the purpose of that study, to count as a mole, the blemish had to measure more than two millimetres in diameter.

Fortunately, when a previously benign mole starts becoming something more sinister or when a new 'mole' appears these are several distinct symptoms. The most important thing to look for is any *changes* in existing moles. The box highlights the danger signals.

MOLES — THE DANGER SIGNS

Size most melanomas are not recognized until they are about 7mm — the size of an old half-penny piece — which is much larger than ordinary moles. Some experts suggest keeping an eye on any moles larger than the circumference of a pencil.

Shape Unlike ordinary moles, which have a smooth regular outline, early melanomas have an irregular shape and a ragged outline.

Colour Early melanomas are irregular in colour, being a mixture of brown or black, while ordinary moles tend to be *either* brown *or* black.

Redness Most early malignant melanomas are inflamed or have a reddish edge.

Bleeding Some early melanomas bleed, ooze or encrust.

Itching If any mole starts to itch, when it never used to, or a new mole appears and itches, then it could be malignant.

'A melanoma caught early enough can be cured with a small operation carried out under local anaesthetic.'

Dr Rhona Mackie

If you have a mole, with any of the symptoms listed in the box, then get it looked at by your GP. It is probably nothing, but as early diagnosis is so important, better to be safe than sorry. This applies to any mole you may have had since childhood, plus any that have appeared since.

In Scotland, there has been a campaign to increase public awareness of skin cancer, with the aim of cutting the country's annual number of deaths (currently 40). Dr Rhona Mackie, Professor of Dermatology at Glasgow University, who was in charge of the campaign, says:

'People don't realize that skin cancer can spread below the skin. Left alone, it will spread throughout the blood or lymphatic systems and reach the liver, the lungs or the lymph glands. On the other hand, a melanoma caught early enough *can* be cured with a small operation carried out under a local anaesthetic.'

She stresses that monitoring has to continue with all skin cancer patients.

The Scottish survey of 180 patients with skin cancer was reported in the *BMJ* and showed that less than a quarter of them went to their GP within three months of noticing suspicious skin changes. Nearly half waited up to a year, while a similar number delayed longer than a year and could have put their lives at risk.

MELANOMAS MISSED BY DOCTORS

However, what is really disturbing is that some GPs are not aware of the risks of skin cancer either.

A fairly shocking report was published in the *BMJ* in April 1986 by a medical team from King's College Hospital, London. Anthony du Vivier, consultant dermatologist, revealed,

> In the past months, we have seen several cases of primary malignant melanoma arising on the face — in which the diagnosis had been repeatedly overlooked — sometimes *for several years by doctors who had seen the patient for other disorders.*

The report was called 'Missed malignant melanomas' and described five different cases including one 37-year-old woman who had had a flat brown pigmented lesion on her face for ten years. During a recent pregnancy, she had seen five different doctors in 14 separate hospital visits and *none* had commented on her facial tumour. It was finally diagnosed by her GP, three months after she had given birth.

By this stage, the melanoma was so large that she had to have extensive plastic surgery to reconstruct her cheek. By the time of operation, the depth of the tumour was over two milimetres and she had been completely unaware of her condition until the diagnosis was made. Earlier diagnosis by any of the five doctors would have ensured a complete cure, but now her future looks decidedly uncertain.

This case, and the four others reported in the area, were all the more terrifying because all the people concerned had malignant melanomas on their *faces,* where they could be clearly seen, not hidden on some other part of their body.

The authors noted that, since skin cancer was no longer rare, doctors should be on the look-out for it, as should patients themselves. It was one thing, they said, to miss something suspicious on the back or back of the calf — where melanomas are commonly found — but quite another to miss something on a patient's face:

> The ultimate aim of health education for malignant melanoma is to reduce the incidence of the disorder by alerting those at the greatest risk — that is fair or freckled people whose skin burns rather than tans (or burns before it tans) to the hazard of recreational exposure to ultraviolet light.
>
> Until such an aim is achieved, reducing the mortality of malignant melanomas depends on recognition of the primary lesion at an early phase in its growth, and certainly before the well-known sinister features of nodules: ulceration, and haemorrage have occured.
>
> As the skin is an organ uniquely readily accessible for inspection and as patients are all too often unaware of the importance of pigmented lesions, all GPs should be alert to the possibility of making a potentially life-saving diagnosis of early malignant melanoma in their patients.

Where public awareness campaigns have been launched, in Sydney, the West Coast of America, Canada and Scotland, doctors have reported larger numbers of people coming forward for confirmation and treatment of *early* skin cancer.

WRINKLES

Skin cancer is not the only bad thing about excessive exposure to the sun's burning rays. These rays break down the elastin and collagen which keeps the skin smooth and supple. Compare the skin on the back of your hand to the skin on your hips, for example (which rarely encounters sunlight), and just look at the difference. One is soft and smooth, like baby skin, and the other is rough and leathery with thousands of 'lacework' wrinkles and crevices. The difference is directly attributable to exposure to the sun.

Doctors in America were so concerned that in the summer of 1985 the Chicago-based American Medical Association's Council on Scientific Affairs issued a special report to alert the public to the dangers of sunbathing in general, and in particular to the current vogue for using sunbeds both at home and in health farms, hydros and beauty parlours.

They confirmed what many of us have already witnessed with our own eyes, particularly among groups of young white women living in hot countries like Israel and South Africa, who look old by the time they are 30:

> 'There is strong evidence that years of tanning will damage the skin and cause it to take on a prematurely wrinkled, weather-beaten, leathery appearance.'
> *American Medical Association*

There is strong evidence that years of tanning will damage the skin, and cause it to take on a prematurely wrinkled, weather-beaten, leathery appearance.

Action spectrum evaluations have clearly shown that UVB is the most carcinogenic (cancer causing) radiation in the ultra-violet spectrum although there are studies that indicate UVA can *augment* the cancer-producing effects of UVB rays.

While skin cancer is largely curable and, with the exception of malignant melanomas, mortality rates usually are low, morbidity rates can be high in terms of disfigurement and scarring.

SUNBEDS AND THE DANGERS OF UVA RAYS

Until fairly recently, it was believed that only the ultra-violet B (UVB) rays were dangerous and that ultra-violet A (UVA) rays were completely undamaging: UVB burned, whilst UVA merely brought the pigment up and tanned the skin.

However, dermatologists are now telling us that UVA is *not* harmless, but instead, penetrates more deeply — where we cannot immediately see the damage because it is long-term. This damage, say the world's leading dermatologists, is irreversible, causes premature ageing, sagging tissue, wrinkles and freckles and will force many of the 18-year-old bronzed beauties on this summer's beaches to be seeking facelifts and anti-ageing potions by the time they are in their thirties.

As most sunbeds use concentrated UVA light it would seem prudent to avoid them if you want to keep your skin looking as youthful as possible for as long as possible. Even the Association of Sun Tanning Operators, which represents people who run suntanning premises in Britain, admits that people with fair or red hair and pale skin who don't tan well in natural sunlight, would be well advised not to use sunbeds at all, even those using UVA.

Even so, sunbed brochures and the staff who run salons offering sunbed sessions will all tell you that their equipment is quite safe and most stress what might well be true, that it is 'safer than natural sun'.

However, what they don't tell you is that until anyone proves otherwise, it is decidely safer to avoid sunbeds altogether. Some sunbed ads even claim that there are other health benefits associated with their use but such claims should be treated with scepticism, if not derision. When *Which?*, the UK Consumers' Association magazine, sent its inspectors out in 1987, they found that 8 out of 9 sunbeds operators were completely unaware of the official guidelines.

Early conventional sunlamps were, of course, far more dangerous than the latest ones, as they emitted primarily UVB rays. Any of us who regularly sat in front of them, especially if we did so without goggles, can not only look forward to a prematurely aged skin, but also an increased risk of cataracts.

Today's sunbeds virtually all use fluorescent lamps which emit about 95 per cent UVA and 5 per cent UVB. Such combinations are quite different from natural sunlight.

British medical authorities have paid little attention to the sunbed craze, and warnings and advice from independent sources are, alas, virtually non-existent in this country.

WARNINGS FROM AMERICA

However, the American Medical Association's 1985 report looked closely at sunbeds, and issued stern warnings against their use. They said:

> Tanning beds and booths are advertised and sold as being safer than earlier types of tanning lamps. Health spas, salons, and 'tanning clinics' frequently advertise 'a safe tan' and 'tan without burning'. Some even advertise their booths as so safe that it is not necessary to wear protective goggles while tanning.
>
> This statement is simply not true, but such claims can instill a false sense of security in those using the newer tanning devices.
>
> Such advertising makes the new tanning devices potentially more dangerous than the older tanning huts because people may be less likely to restrict themselves to short tanning periods.

It is not just the American Medical Association which has shown concern about the use of sunlamps, similar warnings put out by the world's leading dermatological associations have caused the powerful American Food and Drugs Administration to insist that sunbed manufacturers include timers which switch off automatically and that operators provide goggles and insist that they are used.

What happens in individual suntanning salons and at home is of course quite a different matter. For example, in the light of the AIDS scare and the theoretical possibility at least that the AIDS virus can be transmitted through the tear ducts, many people using the fashionable parlours which could be patronized by homosexuals or bisexuals, prefer not to use goggles and risk eye damage rather then the killer disease.

The AMA report on the hazards of suntanning and sunbeds concluded:

> There is no known medical benefit obtained from cosmetic tanning. Exposure to high intensity UVA radi-

ation in the tanning booths currently in vogue is a health hazard.

Nevertheless, there are individuals who decide that the cosmetic benefits of tanning outweigh the potential risks, or, more likely, *do not understand the risks*, and make personal decisions to use a tanning booth, sometimes even in defiance of medical advice.

BEWARE OF SUNBEDS!

'There is no known medical benefit obtained from cosmetic tanning. Exposure to high intensity UVA radiation in the tanning booths currently in vogue is a health hazard'.
American Medical Association

The AMA said it opposed *any method* of acquiring a tan through the prolonged use of UVA and UVB. However, for those who insisted, it made the following *recommendations* which would reduce, but not of course eliminate, the risks:

1 Tanning devices should not be used by individuals who burn easily: those who burn in natural sunlight will burn under a sunbed.

2 Tanning methods should be avoided if there is a tendency to develop cold sores as ultra violet radiation may stimulate production of these lesions.

3 Artificial tanning devices should be scrupulously shunned if medications known to cause photosensitization are being used. These include many antibiotics and antihistamines, some birth control pills, certain agents used to treat acne, some drugs for epilepsy, depression and diabetes, drugs for high blood pressure and certain endocrine disorders. NB This includes a very high proportion of the population.

4 Exposure times must not be overdone. Like natural tanning, artificial tanning must begin with short exposure time. Do not be tempted to prolong the session just because you can feel no burning or because you are paying by the second and the meter has stopped running and you are on 'free time'!

5 Ultra-violet radiation in a tanning booth is so intense that extended exposure can cause serious injury.

6 Protective goggles with blue-grey plastic lenses opaque to ultra violet light should always be used. Simply closing the eyes, using ordinary sunglasses or putting cotton wool over the eyes is insufficient protection against eye damage.

(If you are unhappy about sharing goggles, or feel the ones provided are inadequate, then invest a pound or so in a pair of your own and always use them. The *Which?* report found that one in five sun bed users did not wear goggles and that not all centres insisted they were worn — indeed, some operators even said they weren't necessary.)

7 Ultra violet lipstick should be used whilst tanning.

8 Direct contact with the sunlamp is to be avoided. A handrail should be provided in a booth where the customer has to stand up, and an attendant should always be around in case help is needed.

9 The timing device should never be tampered with and a machine should not be used if it is broken or disconnected.

10 Tell your salon staff about your tanning history and don't be afraid to seek their advice, and go elsewhere if all they are interested in doing is selling sessions and not protecting you against any potential dangers.

SUNBEDS — BIG BUSINESS

Sunbeds are big business. Just how lucrative they can be is shown in this quote from a brochure from Solana Industries Limited, a Swedish company which specializes in sunbeds, sunbed toiletries and other associated 'health' products.

In a club, after the licenced bar and the fruit machines, probably the next most profitable item in terms of cost, power consumption and space is a good quality sunbed.

Yes, for a capital outlay of anything between £1,700 and £3,500, you should at least get your money back in the first six to nine months and look forward to a further three to five years with minimum maintenance.

The brochure then goes on to itemize types of sunbed, together with the running costs and the suggested charges to produce the following profits:

For a *Super 28* model, assuming an average income of £2.50 for 20 minutes (West End salons charge a lot more) and running costs for the same period of 24p:

Profit per month at two hours a day — £231.60.
Profit per month at four hours a day (average) — £463.20.

Profit per month at eight hours a day (maximum) — £1,111.68.

Annually (50 weeks) the figures work out at £2,779.20 if the machine is in use for two hours a day; £5,558.40 if it is in average use of four hours a day, and a staggering £13,340.16 if it is going full blast for eight hours a day.

This clearly a very profitable business to be in, providing you have a popular club atmosphere and a large number of members/clients. I have quoted Solana, but other companies will readily boast similar profit predictions to would-be buyers of their machines.

There are now more than one million sunbeds in use in Europe and the increasing popularity of this form of suntanning has led to moves by the British Standards Institute to introduce safety limits for ultra-violet exposure on all suntanning equipment.

STANDARDS FOR SUNBEDS

It is unlikely that anyone embarking on a course of sunbed treatment will challenge the operators waiting to take their money about the safety of their machines, but if they do feel inclined to do so, all they need ask is whether the machine complies with BS3456. If it does not, the chances are the salon will turn such a 'bolshy' customer away, fearing they might be spying for the Department of Trade!

According to the Association of Suntanning Operators (ASTO), which represents the people who operate this equipment commercially, the new standards are still not tight enough to protect the public.

In particular, ASTO would like to see tighter limits on the use of UVB in sunbeds, particularly those which boast 'quick tans'. These often have fluorescent lights which look like the UVA sunbeds and it is very hard for the customer to distinguish which beds are 'safer' than others.

ASTO suggests that people using health clubs and tanning parlours should ask the operators what the level of UVB output is, and if the operator doesn't know or says that the beds are of the high UVB 'Quick Tan' type, customers should go elsewhere.

ASTO says:

Sales literature and advertisements, especially for imported equipment, often do not state that the UVB output is high. Be sure to purchase or use only lamps with a UVB percentage of 0.5 per cent or less.

All manufacturers will state this clearly on their literature as it is a claim they are proud to make for their *safe* products.

Because of the vast amount of confusion about sunbeds and suntanning, manufacturers, distributors and operators of this equipment decided to set up a Sun Tanning Advisory Bureau in London through ASTO. Advice is available either in their book about suntanning and ultra-violet light or on their telephone number: 01 228 6077.

Amongst other things, they stress that a suntan obtained through sessions on a sunbed does not protect the skin from burning when exposed to natural sunlight. The tan is purely cosmetic, all that it does is create the first layer so that subsequent exposure darkens your skin more quickly. The *Which?* report recommended that people should *not* buy sunbeds, and it did not favour hiring them in case it led to cramming too many sessions in 'to get your money's worth'.

Finally, if despite all my advice and that of the experts, you are determined to go on using these 'electric beaches', then look out for the 'ASTO' symbol, which at least ensures that the centre is following the official guidelines laid down by the Health and Safety Executive.

SUNBED SUNTANNING CREAMS

Since the explosion in the number of regular sunbed users, a whole new generation of suntanning products designed specially to aid a tan and protect the skin from the UVA rays has come on to the market. It is important to remember that these products do not protect the skin against UVB at all, so they should never be worn as an ordinary suntanning product in natural sun. The logic behind using protection against rays that you have chosen (and paid) to be exposed to is very strange, but if you're going to lie on a sunbed, any protection is better than none.

Some companies are beginning to realize the importance of protecting the skin against UVA rays in *natural* sunlight and are developing new products with this in mind. These would not be strong enough for lying on a sunbed. 'Many products with sun screens only protect against UVB rays which cause sunburn,' says Dr Gary Dugan, director of skincare research and development

---

Do not use sunbed suntanning creams in natural sun. They provide *no* protection against UVB rays.

at Avon in America. 'But it is the UVA rays which penetrate deep below the surface of the skin where new healthy cells are forming. These rays break down the support fibre network of collagen and elastin, causing sagging and wrinkling of the skin years later.' As a response to this, Avon brought out *Age Protection System*, which was designed as an 'advanced solar shield complex' — rather like sitting in the sun with a physical barrier in front of your body!

PROTECTING YOUR SKIN AGAINST THE SUN

'Suntanning is a national epidemic', says Leonard Lauder, son of Estée, and president, chief executive and heir to the Estée Lauder company. His company is one of the hundreds which make suntanning formulations which promise either to give you a prettier tan, or to protect your skin completely from the sun's harshest rays, whilst promoting a 'healthy' glow.

The market for suntanning products has been growing at 20 per cent a year for the last decade or so, with sales worth $250 million a year in America and £39 million in Britain. The market was only created in 1936, when the first suntanning lotions for the newly fashionable suntanned look were made by L'Oreal. Their original *Ambre Solaire* is still the best-selling brand.

The market is fiercely competitive, and the campaigns to persuade us to buy a particular brand are concentrated in late spring and early summer to influence the choice of the 50 per cent of women and 30 per cent of men who intend to buy a bottle or two of the product.

About 83 per cent of the products purchased claim to 'aid suntanning', whilst about 12 per cent are 'after-sun' products. Despite all the warnings about the dangers of the sun, only 5 per cent of the population plays safe with fake tan creams.

No suntan product makes anyone tan faster than they would without using it, (unless it contains an accelerator) but an effective product should allow you to stay in the sun longer without burning.

A suntanning product has to be especially safe for use on the skin because it is generally used by all ages, and by people taking all sorts of drugs and in various states of health. Also it is designed to be used repeatedly, several times a day, unlike practically any other cosmetic product. You should also be careful about what skin creams you are wearing when you go out into the sunlight. Professor Malcolm Greaves, Dean of the Institute of Dermatology at St Thomas's Hospital in London, wrote a letter to *The Times* in the autumn of 1987, warning people to be careful when sunbathing so-called 'anti-ageing' cream. 'Users need safeguarding, since they cannot assess the risks and benefits of these preparations, advertising claims for which go far beyond those expected of a cosmetic. The loophole should be closed and these potent drugs brought under statutory surveillance,' he urged. 'My worst fear is the preparations which claim to achieve cell renewal which might be used by people who do a lot of sunbathing. The combination of sunlight and these products might very well induce cancer.'

In a separate warning, dermatologist Dr Vinay Dave of the Manchester Skin Hospital, said that coconut oil, an ingredient in many suntanning products, had been found to cause a bleaching and speckling effect on some skins. He advised sunbathers to leave coconut oil where it belongs — in the kitchen.

SPFs — WHICH ONE FOR YOU?

Different products contain varying amounts of sunscreen and in the late 1970s, a system was developed by the cosmetics industry — in particular the Plough Corporation, which make *Coppertone*, etc. — for labelling suntanning creams with Sun Protection Factors (SPF). SPFs are graded from 1 to 23. Most are between 2 and 10.

The highest number is effectively a total sunblock, allowing one to stay out in the sun for 23 times the length one could ordinarily, before you start to burn. This kind is suitable for the sensitive skin types who go lobster-red within moments of sitting in bright hot sunshine, and who never 'tan'. The lowest SPFs are for those who never burn, mostly those with deeply-pigmented, dark brown skins.

Unfortunately, there is no uniformity of SPFs among the dozen or so leading manufacturers, so you just have to be guided by the blurb on the tube or packet. If in doubt, go for higher SPF than you think you need. You'll still get tanned, even underwater or sitting under an umbrella on the beach, because sunlight is reflected, but you shouldn't burn, which is what all these products are designed to prevent.

American SPFs have higher numbers but tend to give lower protection than European products. For example, people with pale skins and red hair would find they could be pretty safe from sunburn, even in the desert, if they wore a product like Estée Lauder's sunblock cream which has an SPF of 23. This figure is probably equivalent to a British SPF of 15.

You can reduce the SPF level as you build up a gentle suntan, but *remember that dermatologists consider any product with an SPF below 4 probably not worth bothering with.*

CHOOSING A SUN CREAM

No one with a pale skin should go out into strong sunshine without wearing an SPF of 5 or more. In tropical climates, dermatologists say it is foolish for anyone to go out in the sun wearing an SPF any lower than 8.

● Look for descriptions and ads which talk of the dangers of sun exposure, and the protection afforded by the cosmetics you are about to buy.

● Spend money on good quality products *only* if they contain UVB and UVA filters, and have high SPFs.

Use a waterproof suncream even if you are not planning to go near the water, because the skin sweats in the sun and the moisture in sweat — especially if you mop yourself with a towel — removes the protective layer of suncreen you *think* you are wearing. 'Waterproof' suncreens have been tested to withstand half an hour's heavy sweating. Incidentally, the salt in sweat and the sea dissolves a sunscreen more slowly than unsalted water, as in swimming pools.

Professor Albert Kligman, who advises anyone who cares about their skin to stay out of the sun as much as possible, reckons that while an SPF of 2 might absorb about 50 per cent of the dangerous UVB rays, SPFs over 6 absorb 90 per cent.

To work out your own needs in terms of SPFs, consider carefully how long you can sit bare-skinned in strong sun without burning. If it is 15 minutes, an SPF of 6 would allow you to stay in the same sun for 90 minutes without burning.

Some suntan manufacturers sell 'double packs' with different SPFs so you can vary the protection you use according to how tanned you are already and the intensity of the sun. Check that you're getting good value for money, and not merely buying two lots of suncreams without the benefit of any price reduction for sticking to the one brand.

A VARIETY OF PRODUCTS

Sun products vary from, at one extreme, total sunblock barrier creams, which include zinc oxide, to suntan oils which fry the skin as effectively as in a frying pan.

The most effective and cheapest sunblock is zinc and castor oil, which is very popular in some ski resorts and on the beaches of California and Australia where the sun is very strong. It is highly fashionable there to go around with a white nose or lips — or with brilliant 'day glow' colours. In other places you may feel that a blob of thick white or coloured cream on your nose can look unsightly, silly and very unsophisticated — however effective it is (which just goes to show what a strange business fashion is).

Since most oils, including olive oil, coconut oil and baby oil, offer no protection at all, only people with dark skins or very tough non-burning skins should use them.

Most suntan manufacturers make a wide range of products to ensure that they have something for everyone. For example, Schering Plough (the giant pharmaceutical firm which owns *Coppertone*), recently advertised its *Ultimate Sun Oil* from *Tropical Blend* promising: 'Now nothing can come between you and the sun except nature's own moisturizers.' This ad actually boasted that the product contained no sunscreen and recommended its product for those who already had a good base tan, to 'capture the savage tan', which is depicted by showing an oily darkly-tanned girl lying on a beach with a tiger reflected in the sand. But at the same time, the company ran another advertising campaign in which a worried father was holding a bottle of *Shade* over his wife and daughters to deflect the 'bad' rays so that nobody would fry on the beach! (The same company also makes the fake tans *QT* and *Sudden Tan*.)

BEST-SELLERS

The British are the second biggest users of suntan products in Europe, beaten only by the skin care/suntan-crazy French. After the extensive French range of *Ambre Solaire*, which is bought by 25 per cent of sunworshippers, Avon, surprisingly, sells the next most popular brand. Joint third are *Bergasol* and *Nivea* which have held on to their popularity, followed by *Hawaiian Tropic* and Boots' *Soltan* range.

Ambre Solaire is popular in France, but so, too, is the Swiss *Piz Buin*, produced by Ciba, the giant pharmaceutical company. The biggest European seller is said to be *Delial*, according to its manufac-turers, the German pharmaceutical firm Bayer.

A poor British summer usually means that shopkeepers end up with surplus stock on their shelves and bargain hunters can stock up on this years's products during the sales as suntan lotions and oils have a long shelf life.

WINTER SUN

Strangely enough, the industry sells us most of their suntanning products in the winter months while all those holiday ads are being shown on TV and most of us are dreaming of baking hot days and vast sandy beaches as we hug the radiators and sink deep into our winter woollies!

There is also a growing market among the winter sports enthusiasts, because the combination of sun, high altitude and dazzling white snow can be more deadly to the skin than summer sunshine on the beach. Day-long exposure to a combination of biting cold, icy winds, dry air and exceptionally strong UVA and UVB rays can damage unprotected skin. This is because at high altitude, where most wintersports take place, the UVA rays penetrate the atmosphere more easily and reflect off the whiteness of the snow; simultaneously, the UVB rays are more scattered.

The lips are especially sensitive to the sun, because they contain hardly any melanin, the body's natural sunscreen, nor any sebaceous glands to release oil and keep them moist. Extensive burning of the lips can lead to lip cancer, so always use a strong sunblock to prevent any damage when skiing.

CHILDREN AND SUN

In 1986, the American Archives of Dermatology carried a report of a study which showed that if children were persuaded to wear a sunscreen with an SPF of 15 when playing in the sun, and throughout the first 18 years of their lives, they could reduce their chances of developing skin cancer by nearly 80 per cent.

Because sunburn and skin ageing

would also be substantially reduced, the researchers at Harvard Medical School in Boston recommended that doctors advise parents to apply sunscreens to their offsprings' skin as a regular routine.

It should be superfluous to say that babies, who have very sensitive skin and who cannot move out of the sun or roll into the water when they get too hot, should *never* be left in the sun. Unfortunately, however, it is becoming increasingly common to see deeply-tanned babies. If parents are not moved by the idea of the discomfort their babies will almost certainly have to suffer in pursuit of this absurd status symbol, they may perhaps be influenced by the thought that they are laying the foundations for a prematurely aged skin and possible skin cancer.

> Keep babies *out* of the sun!

ACCELERATORS

Several suntanning products contain an 'accelerator' which magnifies the burning rays of the sun and therefore speeds up the rate at which you acquire a tan. They do this by temporarily increasing the sensitivity of the skin to the sun's rays.

Never use a product which contains an 'accelerator' because it can lead to burns, rashes and even skin cancer. Doctors are very worried indeed about the long-terms effects of these products on the skin.

One of the first companies to introduce the idea of accelerators was the manufacturer of *Bergasol*. This contained oil of bergamot — a citrus fruit extract known chemically as 5-methoxypsoralen. Some cosmetic chemists believe that this is extremely damaging to the skin because laboratory experiments on furless mice have shown that it accelerates skin cancer when exposed to ultra violet light.

Although the name suggests that *Bergasol* contains oil of bergamot, it is very hard indeed to find out if this is still the case. My letter of enquiry, sent to the company's headquarters in France never received a reply or acknowledgement. The label is similarly unhelpful, stating only that the product contains 'citrus essence', which could, of course, mean bergamot. Eventually, after persistent enquiries, I found out from the company that *Bergasol* still contains bergamot, but that this has now been 'de-activated', with the active ingredient, bergatnen, over which questions had been raised, having been removed in 1985.

As a rule, I would steer clear of any suntanning products which state on their labels that they contain mysterious 'tropical fruit essence' or similar sounding hyperbole. Who wants to fry or frizzle in the sun, unwittingly basting in some potentially carcinogenic concoction?

A very similar chemical to 5-methoxypsoralen can be used in conjuction with ultra violet light to treat psoriasis. However, the connection between skin cancer and 5-methoxypsoralen is so well established that although psoriasis is a distressing skin disease, this effective treatment is withheld by large numbers of doctors simply because of the risks of skin cancer and patients who insist on having the treatment are fully warned of the consequences.

Warning

Never use a product which contains an 'accelerator'. It can lead to:
- burns
- rashes
- skin cancer

It has not been proved that tanning accelerators are harmful to humans, only a scientifically controlled study could do that. Unfortunately, and perhaps surprisingly, no work is currently being carried out in this area. Future victims of skin cancer might usefully be asked by their doctors what suntanning creams (if any) they used to use.

Most manufacturers of tanning products do not at present intend to remove 'accelerators' from their products because they do not regard the skin cancer risk as a significant one. They argue that, since exposure to the sun carries a risk of skin cancer anyway, anything which accelerates a tan and which therefore might reduce the amount of time a person spends in the sun, could be positive help. This argument doesn't carry much weight, and it seems more likely that people will spend *more* not less time in the sun if they are wearing suncreams they believe are protecting them.

The Association of Sun Tanning Operators issued a warning in 1983 against the use of 'accelerators', when used either in natural sun or on a sunbed.

The association's General Secretary, Frances Allwright, said:

It's crazy to use such a product just for a quick tan. A genuine accelerator works by increasing the skin's sensitivity to sunlight — so it's very easy to burn, even on a sunbed. The long-term disadvantages are much more serious. The ingredients which cause accelerated tanning have been observed to cause marked thickening and ageing of the skin and they may even cause cancer if used regularly over a period of time.

She added that the association's members had stopped using them as soon as the dangers had been pointed out to them. 'But we are very concerned that they continue to be sold and *no one* is alerting people to the serious potential hazards.'

Just to hammer home the point once and for all — do remember that doctors advise people taking drugs which are known to increase sensitivity to the sun not to overdo the exposure or mix the two, so it clearly makes sense not to ignore this expert knowledge, especially in the pursuit of something so trivial as a suntan. If you are planning to sunbathe and are taking prescribed drugs, check with your GP or pharmacist to ensure you will not be at risk. Most forms of contraceptive pill and some antibiotics are examples of drugs which may cause an adverse reaction to the sun.

Other products, often confused with accelerators are *pre-tanning* lotions designed to prepare the skin for sunbathing, the result supposedly being a quicker, better tan.

The criticism of the pre-tanning formulas is that they don't work. Or, as Frances Allwright of the Association of Suntanning Operators says:

As far as I know, not one of these companies has been able to justify their claims as far as the Advertising Standards Authority is concerned.

Added to which, if the suntan lotion manufacturers were able to make products which speeded up the development of a suntan, these would have to work more than skin-deep, making them a drug and not a cosmetic, and they would then run into difficulties with both the Department of Trade and the Department of Health's Committee on Safety of Medicines!

Photobiologists seem to think that the suntanning creams containing alleged 'pre-tan formulas' on sale in Britain are safe, if ineffective, but ASTO warns that you can still buy suntan lotions abroad which contain the old-fashioned kind of accelerators which can be harmful.

Since none of these products is fully labelled, and the industry is particularly secretive about its magical 'pre-tanning formulas', I personally would not risk buying such products on the basis that if they do work, they are not a good idea and are potentially dangerous and if they don't, why waste your money?

FAKE TANS

I said earlier that there was a safe alternative to lying in the sun and that I didn't want to be a killjoy, so here's my advice. Since most people look better with a suntan — fake it!

Once you discover a good fake tanning product, you'll wonder how you could have wasted all that time and money and risked so much damage to your skin and health by sunbathing to get a 'REAL TAN'.

Fake tans are a wonderful invention, giving you an attractive golden colour which slowly washes off, yet manages to fool even your closest friends into thinking you have 'caught the sun'. As Guerlain, the French cosmetics company says in its *Teint Doré* sales brochures, 'Who needs the sun?'

Fake tans have improved a great deal in recent years, although the cheaper ones still have a tendency to turn you a nasty and unconvincing shade of orange. Test a little first on your arm to see how the chemicals in the dye react with those in your skin and what colour it will turn you — it usually takes a couple of hours. But in that couple of hours you can look as healthy as if you'd spent a couple of weeks on the beach, and your skin will be vastly better off in the long run. If you don't do a skin test and the colour turns out to be wrong for you, the fake tan will wear off after a day or two, or a good rub with a facial scrub or a loofah will get rid of most of it.

Problems have been noted with some products containing dihydroxyacetone, (DHA) which is used in most fake tanning products, because it can occasionally give patchy results. But, after nearly 30 years on the market, no long-term damage has been observed.

Some ordinary suntanning products also contain a fake tan, but these are not a good idea as a fake tan has to be applied uniformly and lightly at first, to see how the colour takes, whilst a sunscreen will have to be constantly re-applied and often more so on places like your nose and shoulders where burning is most likely. You could end up looking very peculiar and patchy if you use a combination product in this way! However, such products may be useful for fair-skinned people who want to look tanned and for whom natural suntanning is impossible, and for whom protection is essential whenever they expose their skin to the sun.

Some after-sun lotions contain a fake tan too, and these are not so bad as long as you only rub the cream in once and again make sure it is evenly spread. But, again, you may need more moisturizer than colour so it is best to use the products separately.

You should realize that the brown colour a fake tan gives you will not protect you from sunburn and you should still apply a sunscreen if you intend to sunbathe after dyeing your skin with a fake cream first.

You should always wash your hands carefully after applying a fake suntanning product and be careful when applying it on elbows, knees, ankles, etc. where it may get lodged in creases and give a streaky effect.

Fake tans come in all varieties: creams which stain for a few days, lotions which add a tint (like Guerlain's *Teint Doré* or Boot's *Skin Tint*), or 'body make-up' which is like foundation cream for the arms, legs, and torso. There is also *Ultraglow*, a rather expensive dark powder which gives a good colour to the skin when applied with a large brush, but this is only really suitable for the face, neck and, perhaps, the shoulders.

On the whole the cheaper creams tend to produce less convincing colours, so you may find that this is one case where it is better to buy the more expensive products. I have seen good results with Clarins self-tanning milk (which contains DHA and a UV filter).

While the fashion continues for a golden tan, certainly in summer, and, preferably, all year round, fake tanning creams would seem to be the most sensible way of getting one. Either that, or a very good sunscreen with a high SPF, but, in a typical British summer, you could end up looking lily-white rather than golden brown.

It may be hard to give up sunbathing but you should certainly try — unless you promise yourself to be vigilant for early signs of skin cancer and realize that, in 20 years' time you may be putting your holiday money into the bank account of a good cosmetic surgeon for the facelift you'll need.

A FAKE TAN

- Spread it evenly on the skin.
- Apply sparingly on elbows, knees, ankles or anywhere where the skin is rough or wrinkled.
- Immediately after application the brown colour is liable to come off on sheets or clothes.
- Wash your hands after applying it.
- Reapply regularly.
- *A fake tan will not protect you from burning. You must wear a sun screen too.*

TANNING PILLS

Until recently, it was possible to buy sun-tanning pills, which were usually advertised in the small ads in newspapers. A full course was quite expensive, up to £20, although some companies did offer refunds for unsatisfied customers.

In general, pills which dye you from the inside are not to be recommended because of questions concerning the long-term safety of those containing the active ingredient canthaxanthin. They were banned first in Australia, then in America, West Germany and Norway, and finally, after much deliberation, by Britain in January 1987.

Consumer research in Australia showed that the main reason people gave for using any of the 14 alternative fake tanning products available was the very realistic fear of skin cancer.

Tanning pills like *Orobronze* contained the tanning agent canthaxanthin, a chemical dye simlar to that found naturally in carrots. It is sometimes used as a food additive, for example, to improve the colour of farmed salmon, but then in much smaller quantities than is found in each tanning pill.

Aquatan claims its dye is *naturally* derived from carotene and as yet, no one has questioned the safety of such an ingredient. *Bronzeen* stopped using canthaxanthin in its tanning pills after its original formula was withdrawn by the Australian government. It remains to be seen if suntanning pills will remain now that the manufacturers are now prohibited by law from using canthaxanthin.

You 'tan' by taking the pills every day so your skin turns a yellowy or coppery brown, with the final colour depending very much on your individual skin tone and chemicals. The unabsorbed excess chemical passes through the body and can have the disconcerting effect of turning the faeces brick-red. Although this can be alarming, the customer is warned of this possibility in the instructions and of the chances of the palms of the hands turning orange if too many pills have been taken. Once you stop taking the capsules, the dye starts to fade and disappears after about two weeks. The colour should take effect within three weeks without the sun but much quicker with it.

The accumulation of the dye in the liver and kidneys, together with the yellowish skin colour and the reddish colour faeces could lead to dramatically wrong diagnoses of things like jaundice unless the individual concerned tells the doctor what he or she has been taking. There would not be too much problem about this in Britain, but most people who use tanning pills start taking them (as recommended in the instructions) before they go abroad on holiday, and there have been a few cases of very confused foreign doctors.

Warnings about tanning pills were issued in Britain by the *Drug and Therapeutics Bulletin*, in 1983:

> There have been no long-term studies of extended exposure to quantities greater than those used in food colouring . . . it is disturbing that a new chemical used systematically should be introduced widely without proper monitoring.

Orobronze was made by Laboratoires Applipharm, a French company, although the dye itself was made by the pharmaceutical giant Hoffman LaRoche. The company's spokesman claimed in 1986, before the ban came into effect, that its own studies had shown it to be safe and effective. As it helped people to avoid the dangers of sunbathing, the company claimed that it had even been recommended by cancer charities in Australia. This extraordinary claim was refuted when Su Noy, co-ordinator of information services at the Anti-Cancer Council in Victoria told the Australian Consumers' Association, 'We're not in favour of these products. They encourage people to think it's healthy to have a suntan and lure people into thinking that because they have a tan, they have protection in the sun.'

When I published the medical warnings in the *Guardian* in the summer of 1983, the company's British distributors made a huge fuss and accused me of 'scaremongering'. Their tactics clearly paid off for I saw no other reports questioning tanning pills. (However, nor did the company take the matter any further with the *Guardian*.)

Although all tanning pills are classified as a cosmetic because their effects are purely aesthetic, many experts say that, as they operate more than skin deep, they ought to be called drugs and therefore be subjected to full controls.

Germany banned tanning tablets in 1985 after a survey at Düsseldorf University Clinic found that 19 out of 29 patients who had taken tablets containing canthaxanthin had golden crystalline deposits in the inner layers of the retinas of their eyes. This finding was confirmed in similar studies in Canada, where 12 per cent of tanning pill users had been similarly affected, and in Sweden where reduced night vision and a reduced ability to adapt to changes in light were also noted.

As yet, the long-term effects on normal vision have not been studied. When the British ban was announced, the Department of Trade and Industry stated:

> Sun-tan pills containing canthaxanthin can cause deposits of yellow particles in the retina of the eye which can interfere with twilight vision, dark adaptation and susceptibility to glare. Also the possibility of more

serious damage to eyesight cannot be ruled out.

Although full data was not available to government safety experts, they felt that the information they already had was enough to justify the ban and so the companies concerned were ordered to stop selling their products.

There are four reasons why I have devoted so much space to this product, although it is theoretically no longer available:

1 To remind you that cosmetic products can be put on the market without being tested in the same way that drugs are, and that it is wise to be *very* wary of any new fads.

2 Even the government was fully expecting that other cosmetics manufacturers might be tempted to fill the gap by marketing new suntanning pills, as there is clearly a demand for them.

3 The ban was practically ignored by the media — the only reference I heard was that it had been mentioned on the Jimmy Young radio programme.

4 The long-term effects have not been studied and past users might like to know the facts as they stand.

For example, the possible effects on the developing foetus were never considered. Although the Consumers' Association warned Australian users, 'As with any untested product, we strongly advise pregnant women or mothers who are breastfeeding not to take tanning pills,' most tanning pills did not give such warnings. They passed the buck by advising customers to tell their doctors if they were pregnant or breastfeeding, but such doctors did not have access to any 'contra-indications' because studies had never been done.

Finally, cosmetics are kept by most of us for years, so if you have any tanning pills left over, throw them out!

CHAPTER TEN

MAKE-UP

When most people think of 'cosmetics', they think of make-up, rather than anything else, simply because make-up is the most obvious form of artificial decoration we use.

LIPSTICK

Lipsticks are a blend of oils, fats and waxes used to store a colour—the main selling-point of the product. The base material used has to have a melting point high enough to prevent it becoming soft at room temperature, but low enough to allow it to be usable. The most popular variety is the twist-up form. Used cleverly, lipstick can make thin lips appear more generous, broad ones finer and shapeless ones more shapely.

A greasy base helps keep the lips moist and seductive-looking and it also has the added benefit of acting as an emolient, which prevents chapped and cracked lips. Lipsticks often contain lanolin (to which many women are allergic), petroleum jelly, silicone wax or even castor oil (despite its unpleasant taste!). Perfume, to which women can also be allergic, is usually included, mainly to mask the odour of the fatty base.

Perfumes which taste as well as smell nice are obviously a good idea, although definite fruity flavours have not been commercially successful despite several attempts to introduce them. They have a certain appeal for very young wearers of make-up however, tasting more like sweets than cosmetics.

Unfortunately, in some women, certain lipsticks actually cause a drying and cracking of the lips, known as chelitis. One study showed that this reaction occurred in as many as 9 per cent of users. The ingredient usually responsi-

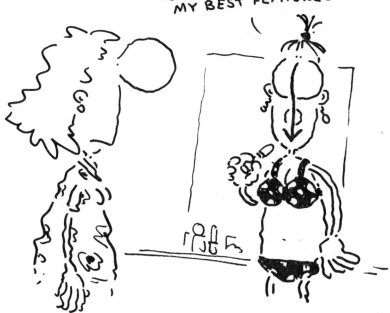

ble is eosin, one of the most common pigments used for staining.

Because of this, certain colours have now been prescribed by the regulatory bodies and the industry has been served with a list of 'permitted' colours for use in all cosmetics, including lipsticks.

However, there is no international agreement on these, so that whereas the colour FD and C Red No 2 is banned in America, it can be used in EEC countries.

Chemicals like titanium dioxide—a white pigment—are used to make pink shades and opaque finishes. If no colour is required, but just a natural moist sheen, lip-glosses or transparent lipsticks are offered. These contain no pigment but have just as many other ingredients. Lip-salve formulations are very similar to these lipsticks, but they usually contain no colour, the object being to keep the lips moist rather than to decorate them.

LIPSTICK DYES

Strong stains in lipstick will penetrate the skin and enter the body. If this worries you, choose lipsticks with little staining power (usually the cheaper brands).

The colour in lipstick has to be strong enough to stain the skin of the lips, to last a long time and to withstand additional moisture from drinking, licking the lips, or kissing. Most forms of eating will wear off lipstick and since it is ingested in this way, it is vital that the ingredients are quite harmless.

Any lipstick which is strong enough to stain the lips for any length of time does in fact penetrate the skin and enter the body. Although it is very tiresome to re-apply lipstick constantly, and although no toxicity studies of the lipstick dyes currently in use are known, cautious women might do better to stick to lipsticks which have little staining power, which happily usually means the cheaper brands.

Lip colour with identical ingredients to the twist-up sticks can also be bought in palettes, the form favoured by beauty editors and professional make-up artists because, used together with a lipbrush, they are thought to be more versatile. Much depends on the skill and co-ordination of the user.

Lip pencils are usually made of harder materials, simply because of the way in which they have to be stored and applied. When they are blunt, leave them in the fridge for a couple of days before sharpening them, or you will end up with a very small stick, and a lot of gooey lipstick jamming up the sharpener.

EYE MAKE-UP

Because of the sensitivity of the eye, eye make-up is among the most vigorously-tested of all cosmetics. Even cosmetic manufacturers are wary of making products which could result in blindness.

The safety of cosmetics has come a longway since an eyelash dye called *Lash Lure*. It caused a number of cases of blindness and one death in the 1930s because it contained an acid that dissolved the eyelashes and burned the eyeball. Products are a great deal safer today and no manufacturer would dare risk marketing such a hazardous product.

WEARING CONTACT LENSES

Women who wear contact lenses should be especially careful about what eye make-up they use and should avoid mascaras which contain any 'lengthening' fibres of rayon or nylon. They should also put on their make-up *after* putting in their lenses, so that their hands are free of creams and oils and bits of powder which could set up infections. If a lens has to be removed during the day, the hands will have to be clean and it may be necessary to remove make-up and powder from around the eye and re-make-up after the lens has been re-inserted. Some contact lens wearers change their make-up altogether once they abandon glasses— especially if the eyes now look bigger anyway, and just stick to a basic eyeliner or kohl pencil, possibly from a hypo-allergic or simple range. Revlon, Almay, and Elizabeth Arden all have mascara, along with eyeliners, suitable for contact lens wearers. Ask, or look out for the labels. Do note, however, that ophthalmologists advise against using eyeliner or khol inside the eyelid. Some opticians sell special ranges of make-up for contact lens wearers, such as Contrapharm. These eye products contain no powder or loose particles, so infection risks are minimized. Ordinary products will do as well, providing you use the right ones, carefully.

MASCARA

Despite pre-market testing, mascara is responsible for a number of eye injuries, which are usually caused by the clumsy use of applicators rather than the contents themselves.

Nicholas Phelps Brown, ophthalmologist and honorary consultant at the Radcliffe Hospital in Oxford, says:

> I have seen several cases of scratched corneas which have resulted from accidents with these applicators. In one case there was minor but permanent damage with recurrent corneal erosion. But usually with proper treatment these injuries can be healed without loss of sight.

Apart from some nasty reactions involving shampoos, shower gels and other detergents accidentally getting into the eyes, Mr Phelps Brown has also had one case in which a patient had mistakenly put corn remover in his eyes, thinking it was eye-drops because the small bottles were extremely alike. It is worth bearing this in mind if you are buying products with such diverse uses, perhaps keeping products intended for use in and around the eyes in a very specific place, far away from everything else.

Some cosmetic eye drops have caused problems but in recent years these have chiefly involved products sold abroad. One product, designed to make the eyes appear bluer and still sold in France, contains copper sulphate and can cause significant eye damage according to Mr Phelps Brown. He has studied the formulation of Optrex, Britain's most popular brand and found it to be harmless.

Mascara comes in liquid, cake and cream varieties. Because of the potential dangers, artificial colours are not permitted in eye make-up, so only natural vegetable dyes may be used, which is why most mascara is black or brown. For blueish shades, soluble blue oil is used, whilst carmine and cochineal (beetles' blood) can be used for red shades. White pigment, such as the titanium oxide used in lipsticks, can be used to lighten shades, along with zinc oxide. Mascara usually consists of various waxes, together with lanolin and pigment.

Until the 1950s, mascara was widely available only in cake form, which required some skill with a brush. The results were often heavy-handed. Another problem with cake mascara was that, in order to mix it at home, it had to be water-soluble, which meant it easily smudged or ran if the wearer cried, got caught in the rain or went swimming.

In the 1960s the brush wand mascara became popular and has remained so ever since. It provides the minimum amount of mascara per application, already loaded on the brush, with no water or saliva required for mixing purposes. Modern mascaras are invariably made waterproof by the addition of polymer-type materials.

EYELINERS

Eyeliners come in liquid, cake and pencil varieties and are designed to be worn very close to the eye itself. A recent development, started by Helena Rubinstein, is the eyeliner that looks like a felt-tip pen and indeed comes with spare cartridges. Although very elegant to look at, and easy to apply in very thin lines, when, by mistake I got the eyeliner into my eye, the ingredients seemed rather irritating. They are also very expensive and, as yet, have not been copied by the cheaper downmarket companies.

> # HINT
>
> Test eye-pencils on the skin between your fingers to see if they drag when applied.
> Expensive pencils are no better than cheap ones.

Cake eyeliners are very similar in ingredients and consistency to cake mascara and they can often be used interchangeably. A typical dry eyeliner is 60 per cent talcum powder, whilst a typical liquid eyeliner is 40 per cent water, and 18 per cent pigment.

Eye-pencils consist of a waxy type of crayon similar in consistency to lipstick. They should be hard enough to keep their shape, but soft enough to apply without scratching the delicate skin between your fingers — if the pencil drags there it will be too rough on the eyelid area. Pencils should apply colour uniformly and not be brittle, or prone to drying up.

Consumer tests in various countries, including Britain, show that although you can pay as little as 80p (*Rimmel*) or as much as £7 (*Helena Rubinstein*) for an eye-pencil, there is very little difference in the end result. The more expensive ones are just packaged more elegantly.

EYE-SHADOW

Eye-shadow can be matt or glossy, plain or glittery. The inclusion of metallic particles such as gold leaf, bronze or aluminium, make the powder sparkly. Although eye-shadows can be bought as creams, liquids, sticks and powders, powders are the most popular because the others tend to 'crease' as time passes, rather than gently fade.

Powdered eye-shadow is basically the same as blusher, powder and talcum powder, but in different colours. Eye colours tend to be quite intense—so much so that only a gentle dab is usually required. Eye-shadow, like other powdered make up, tends to be long-lasting.

Cream eye-shadows are very similar in ingredients and consistency to lipsticks, and commonly include lanolin, paraffin wax, petroleum jelly, zinc oxide and/or beeswax. They are usually applied with a sponge-tipped applicator which can be an intrinsic part of the packaging.

BLUSHER

Rouge is more fashionably knows as 'blusher' these days and currently favoured colours are not red but pinks, browns and 'tawny' or 'natural' shades.

Rouge is one of the oldest types of cosmetics around and some of the ingredients used today are remarkably similar to those used thousands of years ago, for example, red ochre, cochineal and carmine.

By far the most popular form of blusher is powder, although many cream versions are sold. Powder blushers are identical in composition to ordinary face powder—the only difference being the amount of colour used. The ingredients usually consist of 50 per cent talcum powder—often this is as much as 75 per cent of the product. The proportion of colouring varies between one and six per cent, depending on the finished shade.

Wax-based cream blushers are very similar to lipsticks, and look rather like them, too. Thus many products can be used interchangeably. However, waxy blushers have to be smoothed in with the fingertips for a subtle effect and, for this reason, are messier than the powdered form which needs to be 'dusted' on with a large brush.

The staining materials used in lipsticks are not normally used in the manufacture of cream blushers, because of potential allergic reactions which would be much more pronounced on the larger area of the cheeks.

So although you can use a blusher on the lips, it is best not to use a lipstick, especially one with a deep colour, on the cheeks unless it has been specifically designed to be so used.

Cream blushers are also more difficult to apply than powdered rouge, but the finished effects are more subtle and effective than any other kind. As they contain cream, they also blend more into the skin. The base of cream rouges is usually three-quarters lanolin or petroleum jelly.

Liquid rouge, when applied by skilled hands, is also considered to give a better effect. Although it is impractical for most people, containers with a small wick in the neck make it easier to apply the rouge. The product is mostly water, with alcohol added to aid the drying process.

FACE-POWDER

Face-powder is designed to give the complexion a smooth, even finish that looks soft and fresh and natural, and to hide enlarged pores, excessive shine and any minor blotches and blemishes.

It can have either a translucent or opaque finish, according to the current fashion, but whatever the finish, it should be reasonably lasting, and not allow the natural secretions of the skin to work their way through, making the effect patchy. The materials used to enhance the covering power of facepowders are titanium dioxide, zinc oxide (which has better sunscreening properties), magnesium oxide and kaolin. Zinc oxide is also mildly astringent, antiseptic and soothing—indeed, altogether a rather good thing to have next to your skin!

However the major ingredient in face-powder, used for adhesion, is talc, which usually accounts for around three quarters of the total ingredients. Only the best, most finely ground white talc is used for face powder, the rest being kept for body talc. Talc has to be sterilized and screened for asbestos and even tetanus spores, which can occur in some of the countries of origin. It is produced all over the world: Australia, America, China, France, Egypt, India, Italy, Japan, Norway and Spain.

Face-powder has to be absorbent as well as adhesive. Kaolin, chalk, starch and magnesium carbonate are used for absorbency, but kaolin is perhaps the best as it readily absorbs perspiration. Kaolin is a type of clay, a natural compound, with greater adhesive qualities than talc, which is finely ground chalk. However, it can be harsh and so usually forms only 30 per cent of the finished product.

Starch, in the form of rice-powder, was once a very popular form of face-powder, having very fine particles, and giving a very pretty 'bloom'. However, it tends to cake in humid surroundings, or in the presence of a sweaty skin, and can form an unattractive sticky paste which clogs the pores and accentuates facial hairs, and so rice powder was eventually replaced by the talc. However, the modern cosmetics industry has refined rice starch to such an extent that these early difficulties have been overcome and rice starch is once more being used in face-powder today.

Chalk is also used, but usually not in concentrations of more that 15 per cent because it dries the skin. Again, the industry has refined and produced precipitated chalk which has good absorption and grease-resistant qualities, without the drying effects associated with this product.

Magnesium carbonate is even more drying than chalk, but used in small quantities it makes face-powders nicely fluffy and helps prevent 'balling'.

Powdered silk, made from raw silk, finely ground, is used to add 'bloom' to face powders. Because of its luxurious association, the addition of silk also gives copywriters the chance to wax lyrical about the incredible powers of such face-powders.

Colour and perfume are also vital ingredients in face powder, and both are added in delicate quantitites to give subtle effects. Perfumes have to be checked carefully so that they do not clash with the various ingredients already contained in the formula.

COMPACTS AND LOOSE POWDER

For some years, powder has been most popular in compact form. However, compacts can dry up and crack, or become shiny-surfaced and difficult to use.

For these reasons, loose powder has come back into fashion and, with careful packaging complete with gauze or lint covers, it is not as messy on the dressing-table as its predecessors.

CAKE MAKE-UP

This used to be very popular, largely thanks to Max Factor and the early days of Hollywood where it was based on theatrical grease-paint. The ingredients of cake make-up are very similar to those of face-powder, but with added oils, wax and water-dispersing agents. It is designed to be applied with a damp sponge.

Cake make-up is considered by make-up experts to be fine for younger skins, but too drying for women past their thirties, or women of any age whose skin tends to be dry.

FOUNDATION

For some years now, most young women have not worn any powder at all, merely a light base of foundation, preferring this 'natural' look to the more heavily 'caked' make-up look favoured by their mothers and grandmothers. Unlike face powder which blocks the pores, foundation, with its lighter application and greater absorbency, lets the skin 'breathe'.

This has been a major attraction for modern health-conscious women who have been made more aware of the need to preserve their skins than earlier generations, who were more perhaps more concerned with glamour and high fashion. Consequently, many younger women never use face-powder.

Foundation is essentially an emulsified lotion containing pigments, water and talc, which 'evens out' the complexion. However, when the skin sweats, the foundation wears off and, even without sweating, its covering effects do not last very long.

These are the main types of make-up you can buy, although of course the cosmetics industry is always coming up with 'new ideas', which usually means new packaging and brand images rather than different ingredients. 'New' make-up apears on the beauty counters each season purely to seduce us into casting off last year's colours and spending more money. Changing our make-up and hairstyle are the simplest ways for most of us to look fashionable and in tune with the very latest 'look'. And it keeps the money rolling in for the cosmetics and hairdressing industries.

CHAPTER ELEVEN

WHITE MAKE-UP FOR BLACK SKINS?

Although you might find it hard to believe from the international advertising of perfume and cosmetics, which predominantly shows caucasian models, there is a vast and rapidly expanding market for black and brown skins. In Britain, this has been variously estimated to be worth up to £20 million a year for cosmetics and skin care and up to £50 million if hair care is included.

Some companies, notably Revlon and Avon, have been quick to recognize this and enjoy a large following among non-caucasians. However, Revlon has recently been suffering from a black boycott in America after a leading company executive declared that in the next couple of years the black hair care market would be entirely run by white businessmen and the black companies would be driven out of business.

There is, in fact, a huge black-owned cosmetics industry in America, and it is beginning to spread its influence to Britain. However, British shops like Marks and Spencer and Boots also sell lines of make-up (especially foundation) and hair products which are reasonably priced and suitable for the two per cent or so of the British population who don't happen to have pale pink skin.

All of this is quite recent for, until the 1960s, when black skin came to be recognized as beautiful in its own right, make-up for black people consisted largely of skin whiteners and hair straighteners, in other words products to make them look less black.

HAZARDS OF SKIN WHITENERS

Despite the welcome and growing movement of black pride, these products are still around, and selling well, but from time to time there are alarming reports of the hazards associated with their use.

In 1972, the *British Medical Journal* reported that 40 of the 60 Kenyan men and women suffering from kidney disease in one particular hospital admitted to using a skin lightener. When analysed, this product was found to contain mercury, which is a powerful kidney poison. Mercury can also cause severe liver trouble. Although mercury soap was banned in Britain, as recently as 1985 a London company was fined £300 for selling a skin-lightening soap which contained mercury. The manufacturer claimed the product had been produced for export to Africa only (as if that excused the danger) but the soap was found on sale in Brixton, where it was widely used.

Most skin lighteners now sold contain a bleaching agent called hydroquinone. Strict rules are laid down for the maximum two per cent permitted levels of this ingredient, but when several black women recently complained about the piebald blotchy effects produced by some skin lighteners, the Lambeth Trading Standards Officer decided to investigate. Fourteen different brands of popular skin lightener were purchased and analysed. Of these, three contained more than the permitted levels, whilst eight others did not carry appropriate warnings on the labels.

When Ian Bellerby, the Consumer Protection Officer of the London Borough of Haringey, investigated the black cosmetics market in 1985, he found that more than 90 per cent of all prosecutions for dangers found in cosmetics for black people related to excess use of bleach in skin lighteners, excess lead in green eye-shadow and children's make-up sets, and excess levels of dangerous chemicals in hair straighteners.

The report underlined the main problems:

> The international cosmetics industry produces cosmetics almost exclusively for people with white skins, which are not ideally suitable for people with black or brown skins. If you are not white, then you are restricted in the range and type of products available. Most are imported into this country from America, the West Indies, Asia and the Far East. Many are manufactured by small companies, even cottage industries, which use traditional methods and ingredients, and few have the resources to provide adequate scientific and quality controls, thereby putting users of their products at risk.

Many of the people whose job requires them to monitor the safety of such black skin and hair products feel that the number of potential hazards found in them are unacceptable. Mr Bellerby feels that importers should be made liable for safety testing of their products to ensure that they reach British standards for all cosmetics, and that, if a particular item is the source of a complaint, all stocks should be held while investigations take place.

SURMA—LEAD-BASED EYE MAKE-UP

Where there is a serious problem, the authorities can and do act. They did so in 1986 over an Asian make-up which was found to contain dangerous levels of lead, and which was being imported and marketed here by Asians, for use on children.

In 1985, the Department of Trade made one of its rare gestures towards the cosmetics industry when it launched the 'Surma Safety Campaign'. This consisted of publicity leaflets and posters designed to warn Asians that surma—especially if imported—could contain lead, which was poisonous and very hazardous for children.

Up to 50 per cent of the Asian population are estimated to use surma regularly. It is illegal to sell it in Britain, but supplies are regularly brought in from abroad. The government urged parents to have their surma tested by local councils and to take their children to their family doctor if it turned out that the product they had been using had contained lead. Tests in Nottingham, for example, showed that *some types of surma contained up to 86 per cent lead*. The (then) Minister for Consumer

> ## SURMA DANGERS
>
> Tests on surma have revealed dangerous levels of lead in some brands. Parents should have surma tested by their local authority before using it on their children.

Affairs, Michael Howard, said:

> I recognize that the use of surma is a deeply engrained tradition in the Asian community and I have no wish to stop parents from using it. I am simply concerned to warn them that some surma contains lead, which can damage their childrens' health and even lead to their deaths—and to urge them to have their surma tested to see if it contains lead, and if it does, to change to another kind that does not.

Many Asian and black women, especially older ones, do not wear make-up at all, so they do not have any problems. However, young Asians and blacks want to look like their friends and although these days they rarely resort to skin bleaches, they want products that are reasonably priced, widely available and which will serve their needs. Their skin varies in colour from pale coffee, or a dark suntan, to near ebony black, so the range has to be wide.

Revlon has calculated, for example, that there are at least 33 different shades of 'black', so a range of cosmetics for non-caucasians has to have a wide selection of colours—more so than any caucasian make-up range.

SOURCES OF COSMETICS FOR BLACK PEOPLE

Models like Iman and singers like Sade have helped black women to realize they have their own distinctive beauty which white-skinned people envy and admire. Some, whose success depends on their looks, like Bermudan model Sheila Ming, have to go to shops like Cosmetics A La Carte or suppliers such as Charles of the Ritz which mix foundations, eyeshadows and so on, to order.

The cosmetics industry has been slow to respond to the need for black cosmetics. Over £500 million a year is spent on general cosmetics by the bulk of the population but only a handful of products are made specifically for the three million and more non-caucasians who have to make the best of what they can find in the British shops or from mail order companies like Avon.

Although three million sounds like a large number, it is not of sufficient size to get any of the mainstream cosmetics manufacturers very excited. Perhaps 'size' is the wrong word, for market research suggests black shoppers constitute between 10 and 20 per cent of high street chemists' business. However, their individual and collective wealth is apparently not such that the industry feels obliged to woo them with their own cosmetics ranges. This is extraordinary for an industry which panders to most other needs.

Douglas Da Costa, whose company DDC makes one of the two up-market black cosmetics lines in Britain, *Flori Roberts,* did try selling his products in Harrods but gave up when he realized his potential customers were not coming in to buy. He decided instead to sell through high street chemists and his own shops in black areas, and this policy has been successful, although some black women claim they have to travel from one side of London to the other to obtain the full range of products.

Fashion Fair, which is the leading brand of black cosmetics in America, and is owned by the publishers of *Ebony* magazine, Johnsons, was launched in Britain in 1982. To mark its launch, it flew British beauty editors to Chicago via Concorde and treated them to lavish hospitality which even surpassed the typical extravaganza laid on for such occasions by the cosmetics industry.

Fashion Fair's prices are high—just below Estée Lauder's—and the company's policy is that black customers should not be forced to make do with the cheap and cheerful. Within a couple of years of arriving in this country, the company was selling over £1 million worth of products to black men and women. They also make products for white skins with an 'Ebony and Ivory' theme. They are particularly strong on skin care and found that black girls responded especially well to skin care consultants, as they have a lot of specific problems which were simply not being dealt with by either the mainstream (white) women's media, nor the black media.

The company quickly found it was selling more skin care than make-up (which the customers were able to find with other brands by hunting around) and that the average customer was willing to spend about £15 every three or four months.

It is significant that the mainstream brands which have made efforts to supply products suitable for black skins tend to be the down-market cheaper ones. *Outdoor Girl, Max Factor, Avon* and *Rimmel* all sell well among the ethnic minorities in Britain and there are dozens of Avon reps recruited from ethnic minorities.

Although none of the companies have done any specific research, they are aware of the demand, so that Rimmel for instance, launched their *Dark Colour Collection* in 1983, but supplied it to only five out of 100 of their normal outlets. Boots also brought out a new '*Black and White*' collection as part of their 17 range, aimed at younger consumers. On the whole though, shops with few black customers say there is little point in stocking the line. Yet shops with few elderly customers still stock *Grecian 2000.*

The only independent market research carried out in this area, which was done by Syndicated Data Consultants (SDC) found that 16 per cent of women who use cosmetics buy black brands and, when the survey was done in late 1984, this was worth a quarter of a million pounds a month for make-up alone. A market one would have thought worth serving.

The Haringey report suggested that in areas where there were large ethnic minority communities, other local authorities should follow this example and actively encourage and support any local businessman who wanted to manufacture and market cosmetics and toiletries for this community. It also suggested a national initiative which has so far been ignored.

It is very different in America, where around 12 million black women have come to represent 15 per cent of the cosmetics-buying market, worth some $2.3 billion, of which more than $1 billion a year is spent on hair care alone.

BLACK HAIR

Black hair tends to be very springy, coarse and curly. It is better suited to hot tropical climates rather than damp temperate ones like Britain. As a result, there is a massive market for special products to tame and condition black hair and make it glossy. Many products are sold through Afro-Caribbean hairdressing salons who also promote the latest ideas for styling and straightening black hair.

Perming can be a problem for Afro hair, just as it can be for fine flyaway European hair. Pre-testing is essential to determine what strength will be required to get a perm to hold its shape. It may also need perming more frequently near the roots because the regrowth may be tightly curled and make styling rather difficult.

Afro hair often looks stunning and dramatic when dyed, especially with bright colours or bleaches—however the same precautions apply as with European hair. Afro hair usually has weight or body of its own and lends itself to really imaginative and daring hairstyles, which the salons exploit, along with braiding, plaiting and the sewing or weaving in of extra pieces to lengthen the hair.

BLACK HAIRDRESSING SALONS

Whereas the cosmetics industry serves black-skinned people rather poorly, the hairdressing industry caters rather well for this market, with more than 130 specifically black hairdressing salons in Britain. In black areas of the big cities like London and Birmingham, there is usually a wide choice of establishments, all expert in dealing with the special needs of black hair.

Chemists and hairdressing salon owners have recently been complaining because black hair care products are being widely sold in black areas by all sorts of shops, including grocers and off-licences. Whilst the level of fierce competition may be bad news for the retailer, the resulting amount of choice and low prices seems like an excellent thing for the customers.

However, shops in areas where black people may not live but where they work and shop in their lunch hours, do not seem to realize how many potential sales they are losing.

It remains to be seen whether the two giants, Revlon and L'Oreal, are happy to neglect the potential black hair care market in Britain, or whether they will expand from their successful base in America to offer the same range of products black American people have enjoyed for the last decade or so.

CHAPTER TWELVE

THE NAILS

The finger- and toenails are probably the toughest and most chemically resistant parts of the human body. The nail itself is lifeless and contains no nerves or blood. You can pierce the tip and not feel a thing.

The fingernail is chemically similar to hair—which is also dead—and is composed of a substance called keratin. The nail is a very accurate barometer of a person's health, both physically and emotionally.

Various medical conditions can be diagnosed by looking at the fingernails, including iron-deficiency leading to anaemia, which manifests itself in spoon-shaped nails. Pitted and yellowing nails which lift from the nail-bed are characteristic of psoriasis (or a fungus infection of the nail). A white line or pronounced ridge which grows out indicates a recent serious illness or shock. Lead poisoning shows up in the form of a thin blue line across the nail, while red flecks in the nails can indicate heart disease and rounded over-curved nails can aid the diagnosis of respiratory diseases.

The nail is based on a nail bed which contains blood vessels and nerve endings. The nail grows out from the matrix, which is nourished by the blood supply. At the base is the cuticle, which consists of tissue very similar to the outer layers of the skin.

Because the nails are so tough, the cosmetics manufactured for use on them are relatively powerful and should therefore be used with extreme caution in relation to other parts of the body. Because you use your hands to touch other parts of your body, including sensitive spots like your eyes and nose, you can cause additional skin reactions if you are allergic to the nail varnish you are wearing.

NAIL BITING

This is a very common habit but very little research has been done on it. The reason most people bite their nails seems to be psychological, and like other habits, it is something acquired in childhood and usually, although not always, lost in adulthood. Being away from routines associated with nibbling, such as watching the TV and chatting on the telephone, reduces the amount of chewing.

Two women I know well only gave up biting their nails after they became divorced.

Since most psychologists seem to agree that biting the nails is a sign of anxiety and a method therefore of externalizing one's fears, I personally don't think nail-biting is all that terrible—it is certainly healthier than smoking or drinking, comfort-eating or taking drugs or tranquillizers, for example. All of these have serious long-term repercussions.

Parents often try to stop their children biting their nails by using products like *Stop and Grow,* or the old-fashioned remedy of putting mustard or some nasty tasting substance on the nails. The trouble is that these come off the second you wash your hands and are, in my experience, a waste of time and money. Children who bite their nails unconsciously while watching TV, can sometimes be helped by having a piece of modelling clay to play with—it keeps their fingers busy. Perhaps knitting or 'worry beads' might perform the same function for adults.

Another idea, depending on the sex and lifestyle of the biter, is either to try and wear gloves at times when biting is most likely to take place—for example, when you settle down to watch TV, or when you're on the telephone, or on the train—or to try wearing nail varnish.

The latter may look awful on short unevenly bitten nails, but at least it draws the biter's attention to the nails—which is important as most nibbling is done absent-mindedly. Addicted biters will probably nibble off the nail varnish instead, which may not be very good for them.

However, as all biters will know, once the nail does have a chance to grow, either accidently, or as the result of a deliberate attempt to stop the habit, the tiny unfamiliar white tips are something they become fiercely proud of. Unfortunately, years of biting softens the nails so nail hardeners are a good idea, as are rubber gloves and handcreams.

In my experience, nail-biting is an addictive habit which can only be stopped by a change in lifestyle or stress-levels or something equally significant, and cosmetic treatment is of little use.

NAIL COSMETICS

CUTICLE REMOVERS

These come either in creams or liquids and usually consist of an alkaline solution with added glycerine or propylene glycol. *They are extremely drying and should be used very sparingly and washed off as soon as the desired effect is achieved.* They usually consist of a very powerful alkali—more powerful than those used in hair removing solutions—and are one to five per cent sodium or potassium hydroxide. They are often so strong that they will erode glass and are therefore usually packaged in non-transparent containers which don't reveal erosion from the contents!

There are also cuticle softeners which can be applied before any excessive amounts of cuticle are removed with scissors. They contain ammonia usually. A better and cheaper alternative for most people is to soak the fingernails in warm soapy water—pushing back your cuticles after a long soak in the bath is usually very effective.

NAIL WHITENERS/BLEACHES

These are usually used by professional manicurists to whiten the underside of the tips as well as to remove staining caused either by strong nail varnishes or by things like potato and other vegetable and fruit juices.

If possible, women whose work stains their nails should wear rubber gloves as much as they can to protect both hands and nails. An effective bleach is *Perox Chlor* which like its rivals, is based on hydrogen peroxide.

NAIL HARDENERS

These are frequently used by women whose nails are brittle and prone to flaking or splitting. *Most contain formaldehyde which is known to cause problems such as onycholysis, in which the nails start to separate from the nail bed, or discolouration or haemorrhaging of the nail bed or an allergic reaction on the fingers.*

You might like to replace hardeners by a regime of soaking the nails in olive oil or Vaseline to counter the lack of moisture in the nails which caused the brittleness and flaking. Another alternative is to eat lots of gelatin, as recommended by women's magazines and old wives' tales. In fact, this has some scientific basis and is endorsed by the reputable *Harry's Cosmeticology,* which quotes six studies in which gelatin was found to have had an effect a month after being consumed.

As with most cosmetics, any claims for improvements made by the manufacturers of nail hardeners should be treated with some scepticism as the health of your skin, nails and hair depends on your overall health, not your cosmetics budget.

NAIL VARNISH

Nail varnish is hugely popular and is worn by most women at some time in their lives. Even women who bite their fingernails may take great pride in always having beautifully varnished and pretty toenails. And women who wouldn't dream of using make-up on their faces may discreetly apply nail varnish from time to time. Fashion priestesses and models often say that a woman is not properly dressed unless her nails are immaculate.

A good nail varnish should be easy to apply, not go thick in the bottle, and remain unchipped once applied, without causing any underlying staining or allergy. Provided it is kept out of sunlight and away from direct heat, a bottle of varnish should last a long time.

A new development in 1986 was the launch of nail polishing 'pens', led by Christian Dior, and followed by Cutex. *Living* magazine carried out a consumer test on nail polishes in December that year and concluded that the polishing pens compared badly to traditional nail polish in terms of application and staying power. Most users wanted the new pens to work and this should perhaps encourage the manufacturers and their rivals to work on improving the products.

Incidentally, the *Living* consumer testing rated Chanel's nail enamel the best—unfortunately it was also the most expensive. At the cheaper end of the market, Sally Hansen's *New Lengths Micro-Fibre Strengthener* was found to have excellent staying power, lasting some testers a whole week without chipping, and was considered good value. Mary Quant and Maxi rated indifferently and Revlon was rated only marginally better. And the best that could be said about Yardley's *ESP Stayfast* was that it was very easy to remove!

HINT

All nail varnishes use the same formula, so there is no point in buying an expensive one.

Other consumer research, notably in America, suggests that as all nail varnishes use the same formula, there is no point in buying an expensive one and you should be guided by colour and personal taste alone.

Claims by some manufacturers that their nail polishes also condition the nails should be taken with a handful of salt. Like any other cosmetic, polishes are superficial—they have no effect on the internal keratin structure of the nail, they merely coat the surface.

NAIL VARNISH REMOVERS

These usually contain acetone, glycerine and possibly a perfume. Like cuticle removers, they are very drying and should be used sparingly. Some of the more expensive products replace the acetone with ethyl acetate, which is less drying. Some claim to be conditioning, but any substance strong enough to remove enamel cannot be good for your nails and so removers should be used as sparingly as possible. If varnish chips off one nail, touch up with more varnish rather than taking the whole lot off with remover and starting again.

These products are highly inflammable and should never be used near heat or by anyone who is smoking. The fumes can be quite overpowering and it is a good idea to keep a room well-ventilated when you are using them. The same warnings apply to nail varnish. These should also be kept well out the way of children who find their colours appealing; cases of poisoning through drinking it are not unheard of.

FALSE NAILS

These are very popular and perhaps the fastest growing section of the nail market. Certainly at the latest 'Salon' exhibition at London's Earl's Court, the longest queues were at the stands offering various false nail services.

False nails can either be built on to the originals, or simply glued on and filed down as a competely false unit. Either way, the real nail continues to grow underneath. Some women are allergic to the chemical composition in some of the acrylic-type nails. The worst thing they can do is to try and cover up an allergic reaction by sticking on false nails and hoping for the best. Once something as sturdy as a nail starts reacting to a chemical substance, stop using it and all others like it at once! False nails should not be used by women who have mis-shapen nails as the results are only as good as the surface to which they are applied. They should also not be worn permanently, or constantly replaced as the nail must be allowed to breathe from the cuticle at some time.

NAIL PROBLEMS

It is relatively unusual for nails to become damaged of their own accord, but the use of cosmetics and manicure instruments can cause considerable damage in some unlucky people.

For a start, many women are allergic to nail varnish, nail varnish removers and cuticle removers. The latter are quite possibly the strongest chemicals used in cosmetics of any kind. Indeed, the ingredients used in nail varnishes are similar to those used in powerful household drain-cleaners!

Once the nails become sensitive, it is usually best to cease using any cosmetic preparations or techniques because they can become much worse. There have also been considerable problems with nail hardeners, especially those which contain formaldehyde.

By far the most common problem, however, is discoloration resulting from the use of certain nail varnish colours, especially very dark reds and bright pinks. This mainly occurs when the varnish is applied directly on to the nail, without using a protective base-coat. The staining which occurs is deep and usually lasts for as long as it takes for the nail to grow out. This is because the pigment 'bleeds' into the nail. Unfortunately, most manufacturers do not warn their customers of these risks and by the time any individual discovers this unattractive reaction, it is usually too late to do anything about it. The only solution is to wait for the discoloured nail to grow out.

A relative of mine experienced just this reaction. After using her favourite nail varnish her nails turned a nasty nicotine-yellow and it looked as if she had become a very heavy smoker. I wrote to the cosmetic company and asked what she could do, pointing out that she had tried using a base coat but that it had not really made much difference.

The reply from the company was cavalier and dismissive and certainly made me disinclined to use their products again. An added insult was that they included a promotional leaflet on their 'new' colours. A more caring and informative reply would have been much appreciated. The company certainly lost my custom and that of my relative.

KEY POINTS FOR NAIL CARE

- Cosmetics used on nails are very powerful—handle them with care.
- Always use a base coat before applying nail varnish. If nails still go yellow, use a different shade.
- Wash off cuticle removers as soon as possible
- Touch up chipped varnish rather than removing it all.
- Try eating gelatine or soaking the nails in olive oil rather than using hardners.
- Don't use nail varnish or remover near a naked flame or in a confined place or in a public place.
- Keep remover away from polished surfaces, plastic baths, etc.
- Don't use false nails on mis-shapen nails or nails showing an allergic reaction. Keep them for occasional use.
- Keep all nail cosmetics out of children's reach.

CHAPTER THIRTEEN
HAIR: A CROWNING GLORY OR A CHEMICAL LABORATORY?

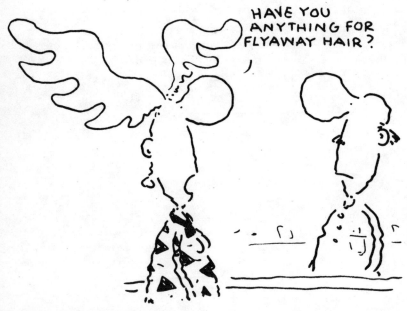

The hairdressing industry, and the beauty magazines, have brainwashed and bullied most of us into thinking that unless we have our hair cut, or at least trimmed, every six weeks, then we'll all end up with frizzy shapeless mops, full of split ends and worse.

It has taken me years to realize that my hair only begins to look good six weeks *after* I've had it cut, or had anything to do with a hairdresser, and my hair always looks its absolute worst the day after I've had it done. I don't know why, perhaps it is the artificial way they part it, and then blow dry it into a style or shape which does not suit the natural weight of the hair, but whatever the reason, I always feel the need to wash my hair as sson as possible and long for it to grow back the way it was!

Victims of the six-week tyranny include a friend of mine who, like many others, has allowed hairdressers to mess around with her hair so much that it has now lost all its natural shape, shine, and bounce. She once returned from the hairdresser with her mousey hair turned bright orange and frizzed into a ghastly mess. A perm had reacted badly with a recent dyeing episode. For days she wore a headscarf and made trips back to the hairdressers while the staff attempted to rescue the disaster. What amazed me then and now, is how this intelligent and attractive girl took it all so calmly. Had this been a business cock-up, or a bodged repair on her car, there would have been legal threats, demands for refunds and all sorts of mayhem. Instead of which, she trekked backwards and forwards, grateful for their attentions, surprised that they were not planning to charge her further (the initial blunder cost her about £30) and above all, it never occured to her to complain to anyone else about what had happened.

Something seems to happen to most women once they cross the hairdresser's threshold. They become passive creatures, apologetic for the natural state of their hair and positively grateful for any havoc that the hairdressers can wreak upon it.

As a student, I used to get my rather long hair cut and highlighted free, by volunteering as a model at most of London's top salons — Leonard, Ricci Burns, Jingles, Trevor Sorbie, etc. The fashion then was for hair to be cut savagely short. Many a time I was passed over by a disdainful teenage trainee stylist, not interested in my 'just a trim' or 'just a bob' request.

I was constantly amazed at how many other volunteers, previously determined to hang onto their beautiful tresses, were trapped into having them lopped off and crudely cut into whatever was the latest faddish look. This may have helped the junior concerned to pass her exams, but did nothing for the poor creature who had to go around for the next few months looking ludicrous.

My stubborness paid off, because fortunately a lot of hairdressers' clients, including leading actresses and models, still wore their hair long, and hairdressers constantly needed to practise on models who still had long hair. Therefore, colleagues over the years have often been surprised to take messages from hairdressers wanting to know if *they* could have some appointment or other with *me*, rather than the other way round . . . because some famous actress was coming in the next day to have her long hair put up and they needed to practise the night before.

Notwithstanding all of this, I do recommend offering yourself as a hairdresser's model, but choose your salon carefully. Go for the best, stick to your guns, and be prepared to walk out if they refuse to cut your hair as you want it . . . and always tip generously, since you will be charged nothing, or only the cost of the materials for whatever you have done.

Conversely, if you are paying for having your hair done, treat the 'service' as you would anything else, such as having your car fixed, and be prepared to challenge the quality of the work or the bill if you think you've been ripped off. Do not be humiliated, put down, or embarrassed by any hairdresser.

If your hair, like mine, looks traumatized each time you visit the hairdresser, either resign yourself to the natural look, or carefully, perhaps with the help of a friend, try and do it yourself, at home.

In July 1987 *Which?* looked at hairdressers and their salons and concluded that, although you might be entitled to a refund or compensation if things went wrong, *proving* carelessness or negligence is very hard. It also pointed out, 'the added difficulty when complaining to a hairdresser may be psychological — it's not easy to be assertive when you really feel like hiding'.

HINT

Save money by offering yourself as a hairdresser's model.
- Choose your salon carefully.
- Insist on having your hair cut the way you want it.
- Tip generously.

SHAPE AND STYLE

Healthy hair is surprisingly strong and elastic. Reshaping it can only be done by softening the keratin in it, and then restyling it before it dries into its natural shape. The easiest way to do this is by wetting it and then styling it before it dries with the help of curlers, rags, rollers, steam tongs or whatever.

Setting lotions and the newer hair gels all help hair to hold its shape, but, depending on the thickness and heaviness of the hair, it will soon fall back into its natural style unless artificially tampered with by chemicals.

The most significant cosmetic development of the 1980s as far as the consumers are concerned has been the development of gels and mousses and other 'sticky' things to slick on the hair and turn it instantly *reversibly* into spikey trendy styles. These styling products have grown so fast that they have doubled their own sales levels each year since they were introduced.

The otherwise health-conscious 1980s saw a comeback for hairsprays, which had been largely relegated to the back-shelves of supermarkets after the back-combed bouffant styles of the 1960s gave way to the shaggy, natural styles of the 1970s.

WARNING

Never use aerosol hairsprays - particularly if you have respiratory problems. They are bad for you - and the environment (see page 210).

However, the American Consumers' Guide to the Cosmetics Industry suggests that you should never buy aerosols:

The most important point to remember in selecting a temporary waving product is *never* buy an aerosol. The health risks of an aerosol spray are enormously greater than a hair-setting lotion or non-aerosol pump hairspray.

The authors insist that hairsprays are a real health hazard, responsible for nearly 400 deaths since the early 1970s. The chief danger, they say, is to the lungs, because the aerosol particles are so fine they penetrate to the deepest part of the lungs where they can get into the bloodstream. People who have respiratory problems, such as asthma, are particularly vulnerable. There is even some evidence that aerosol sprays may be a factor in lung cancer.

This danger was identified over 30 years ago, but of course has been rejected by the cosmetics industry. They argue that tests on animals using aerosol hairsprays have not resulted in lung diseases or death.

Many companies have now removed the fluorocarbons from aerosols and replaced them with what are claimed by the industry to be 'environmentally safer hydrocarbons, such as propane, butane isopentene and isobutane, which are chemically derived from natural gas. Unfortunately, these substances are highly flammable — with a 'blowtorch' effect. Indeed they are so flammable that they are used in cooking, heating and soldering! Despite warnings on the containers, each year there are hundreds of accidents related to the use of aerosols in Britain and America and other countries where they are commonly sold.

PERMS

Modern permanent waves were developed about 20 years ago and were designed to disrupt the hair chemically in order to change its texture and shape. Repeated applications of perm fluids can weaken and ultimately destroy the hair and meanwhile make it brittle and unhealthy.

Various types of hair respond differently to perms — thin fine hair will not hold a perm because it does not have as many fibres as thick hair. Unfortunately, many people with hair like this merely arrange for a stronger — and more damaging — perm the next time round rather than accepting that this is one artificial process they will have to live without.

Hair that has been bleached or dyed has been weakened, and the hair will be much more vulnerable to the harsh chemicals in perms, hence hairdressers' warnings that colouring and perming sessions should not be carried out too close to one another, for fear of the potentially disastrous consequences. If you want to have your perm before going on holiday to a sunny country, do so at least four or five weeks before you go, because the sun combined with the perm will result in dramatic lightening of the hair.

Generally, the more porous the hair, the more waving lotion will be needed.

To make matters more complicated, hair may be unevenly porous from root to the tips, and this has to be taken into account when applying the lotion or uneven, frizzy mops may result:

In the 1950s, many people permed their hair at home, often with fairly dreadful consequences, either in terms of aesthetics, or damage to the hair. Home perms are still sold and apparently used by up to 40 per cent of people who want a perm, but the formulations are a great deal milder than those in salons and results may not be as dramatic or effective. (This is true incidentally, of many hair colours, especially bleaches.)

These days most perms are carried out in salons, by hairdressers, and are usually applied cold in two stages. The first step involves removing the chemically resistent sebum with strong chemicals — including ammonia to soften, swell and break the bonds in the individual hairs. Strands of hair are curled around curlers to provide the required shape. The timing of this stage is crucial in determining how tight or soft the perm will be. The process usually takes 10 to 40 minutes but the hairdressers or individual should carry out frequent checks to see how the perm is 'taking'.

The second step is to apply a neutralizing lotion, usually of hydrogen peroxide, to reverse the effects of the waving lotion by re-forming the bonds into curls or waves. This stage also removes the residue of the waving solution.

The formulations used in perms are very similar to those used in depilatories, so mixing the solutions in the right quantities is vital to avoid the possibility of destroying the hair instead of waving it. It is also essential not to get any of the solutions in the eyes or on the skin, including the scalp. This is especially so if you have any cuts or sores on your hands or skin which might be exposed to the chemicals. It is for this reason that it is important to choose a skilled hairdresser or, if you are attempting to do a home-perm, a careful assistant to help you.

Above all, you should be aware that the main chemical ingredients in perms are extremely poisonous and dangerous. Hairdressers wear rubber gloves and home permers are recommended to do the same. Drops of the solutions spilt on towels or clothes will cause damage. These products should be treated with fear and respect. If accidentally spilt in the eyes, copious amounts of water should be used to wash them out. Left in, these solutions can lead to blindness. Even the tiniest amounts could be fatal if swallowed, so keep them well away from inquisitive children. Incredibly, some mothers perm their childrens' hair

and in my opinion this is unforgivable and totally unnecessary.

WARNING

- The chemical ingredients in perms are **extremely dangerous and poisonous**. Home permers should follow instructions precisely, wear rubber gloves and treat the lotions with the greatest respect. Lotion in the eyes can cause blindness.
- Do not keep home perm materials in the house if you have children.
- Put leftover solutions down the lavatory.
- Do not let teenagers experiment with home perms.

If teenagers insist on having a perm, they should be given every encouragement to go to a salon (as a model if necessary) rather than practise at home. These are dangerous chemicals that they would not be allowed to handle unsupervised at school, so don't let them experiment with them at home just because they come in a pretty, shiny box and are on sale in every chemist in the high street.

Not to put too fine a point on it, the advantage of going to a hairdresser for a perm, rather than doing it yourself, is that you have a comeback should things go wrong. Because the effects are permanent, this is one aspect of the cosmetics industry in which 'doing it on the cheap' is not recommended.

HAIR COLOURING

Many women have experimented at one time or another with colouring their hair at home or having it done in a hairdressing salon. Younger men are increasingly using hair colours, too, and not only the punks. Look closely and see how many men you can find with 'sun-kissed' highlights.

From teens to your final years, you will probably be tempted to tamper with the colour nature intended your hair to be, especially if you are naturally mousey or going grey. There are very few women, apart from Scandinavians, who retain natural blonde hair throughout their lives. This colour hair starts off blonde — even white — in childhood, and gradually becomes a boring shade of nondescript mouse in the twenties, thirties and middle-age. Many famous 'blondes' (for example Britt Ekland, who highlights her hair) are natural 'mice'.

Jean Harlow and Marilyn Monroe started the craze for peroxide bleaching of the hair and to this day many hairstyles are ruined by the sad-looking sight of black roots against bleached white ends.

Since the 1970s, hair colouring has become much more subtle, with most people opting for the more expensive and time-consuming but less obvious 'highlights' than a full change of hair colour.

However, a bleach is still used as the basis for most highlights and can be just as damaging as the old peroxide which used to be left on the hair so long it weakened it.

Unfortunately, highlights need quite a lot of skill, and unless you have a friend to help, it is one of the things which is better left to the professionals. If you volunteer as a model, a head of professionally-done highlights will cost only slightly more than buying a home highlighting kit and trying to do it yourself. The aim is to look natural, and for this you need to get at the back of the head too, which is difficult to do yourself. However, if you really want to try it, it is better to highlight your hair in two sessions — most packs come with two sachets of the mixer-bleach. You can then judge the effect after the first attempt, and make good any patchy bits on the second.

People argue over which method is

best — foil-wrapped or the plastic bag with holes in it. The bag method is more painful, because you, or the hairdresser has to pull the strands through the holes, but on the other hand you can get nearer the scalp so re-growth won't be a problem so soon. The silverfoil leaves a wider gap usually, and takes ages, and is therefore more expensive, but it doesn't hurt as much!

THE DANGERS OF HAIR DYES

Of all the cosmetic preparations currently available, perhaps none have had as many problems and been associated with as many risks as hair dyes. In the mid- and late 1970s there was a considerable consumer campaign in the United States to clamp down on hair-dye manufacturers when it was discovered that many of the chemicals used could cause cancer in animals and might therefore have the same effect on humans.

In 1977, the American National Cancer Institute investigated coal-tar hair dyes and produced a fairly damning report on the industry called *Cancer and coal-tar dyes: an unregulated hazard to consumers*. Amongst other things, it found a total of ten carcinogenic substances regularly used by the manufacturers of various hair dyes.

The upshot of the campaign was that one particular ingredient, 2,4 diamino-toluene (sometimes also known as 4MMPD or diaminoanisole) was banned completely as being too carcinogenic even though *it had previously been used in up to half of all hairdyes on the market*. Several other compounds ceased to be used because of potential risks.

However, hair dyes still tend to be responsible for a high proportion of complaints received by the authorities in relation to burns, rashes and other forms of skin irritations. Yet despite the problems, millions of women and men continue to buy and use hairdyes and tints in vast quantities. Not only that, but they continued to do so during the cancer scare in the late 1970s. The cosmetics industry's representative body in America, the Cosmetic, Toiletry and Fragrance Association, issued soothing reassurances, claiming that the carcinogenic substances were no longer used in hair dyes by manufacturers, yet customer groups and the government monitoring agents continued to find dyes containing such ingredients on sale in many drugstores.

In Britain, the sister industry organization, the Cosmetic, Toiletry and Perfume Association, also insists that hair dyes are safe, according to its General Secretary, Marion Kelly.

One cosmetic chemist I spoke to gave the typical industry response:

> The fact is, people would have to drink about 20 bottles of the stuff every day for about 80 years to produce the same amount of cancer that was found in the laboratory animals. The chance that hair dyes cause cancer in humans is low and probably nor worth talking about, especially as humans knowingly subject themselves to very dangerous carcinogens all the time, for example, by smoking or sunbathing.

A CASE STUDY—NO ACTION TAKEN

In January 1987, the *British Medical Journal* reported the deaths of two middle-aged women in Belfast. The deaths were caused by kidney failure brought about by poisoning from hairdyes, which both women had used for many years.

The suspected substances was para-phenylene-diamine, a common constituent in many permanent hair dyes, used by millions of people every year. The report noted that about one person in 25 is sensitive to this ingredient, whilst about one in 100 are super-sensitive and develop dermatitis or asthma or some other common reaction.

Commenting on the case, Marion Kelly, of the Cosmetics, Toiletries and Perfume Association, merely said: 'This dye has been used for many years and this is the first report we have heard of kidney damage'.

An outcry would have followed such deaths if a pharmaceutical drug had been involved, but there was no call for an investigation, no ban on the ingredient and no action taken by the cosmetics industry. *Not one single magazine published details of the case.*

The overwhelming conclusion reached by both the cosmetics industry and the consumer is that if there is a small risk of acquiring cancer — or kidney disease — through hairdyes, it is a risk most people will take in the interest of beauty and all the benefits that that can bring.

It can no longer be disputed that many chemicals in hair dyes do penetrate the skin of the scalp and thus can enter the bloodstream. The *Archives of Dermatological Research* published a paper in 1985 which showed that up to one per cent of any tested hair dye was absorbed this way.

If hair dye is used regularly and repeatedly, as it was used by the two Irish women, the one per cent can build up over the years into a serious health hazard. And, of course, people who start dyeing their hair usually continue to do so because otherwise their roots show and look unattractive — and give the game away.

What has emerged from all the fuss is that on the one hand, the regulatory authorities have virtually no direct control over what chemicals find their way into hair dyes, and on the other, we now know for certain that such chemicals do enter the bloodstream from the scalp. We do not know what potential harm these substances could do for example, to a foetus, so pregnant women might consider it well worth avoiding having their hair dyed during pregnancy. We also know that because there are so many carcinogenic substances around us, all the time, that it is usually impossible to prove that any particular substance causes a cancer, which normally takes 15-20 years to manifest itself.

I think it is foolish to risk using hair dyes. If your are one of those people who regularly dyes her hair, but considers smoking far too risky, just give it some more thought, and try reading some labels. If you *must* dye your hair, always follow the manufacturer's instructions, including wearing gloves, and be sure to keep the product off the scalp itself. Avoid permanent hair dyes altogether, and avoid those products which carry strong warnings, because the stronger the wording, the more chemically active (and potentially dangerous) the ingredients. Finally, *if you suffer a nasty reaction, report it at once, both to the manufacturer and to your local Trading Standards Officer.*

On the purely cosmetic side, the thing that worries most consumers is the fear that the hair will turn a peculiar and unpleasant colour which, if permanent, will be a major problem. It is possible to get round this by doing a strand test, which though tedious, is worth doing. Simply snip off a sample of your hair and test it separately.

At least one hair dye manufacturer, Warner Lambert, has had the bright idea of bringing out miniature versions of their *Poly* dyes so that consumers can run a sample test first. This seems a good idea and one that will perhaps be copied by rival manufacturers.

As well as permanent dyes, there are also tints and bleaches, which usually contain less chemically-active substances. Most bleaches used in highlighting, for instance, contain hydrogen peroxide which destroys the melanin in the hair fibres, removing the natural colour, just as household bleach will take a stain out of fabrics. Bleaches can be very strong and therefore damage the hair, they can also cause skin irritations. The better bleaching products contain conditioning materials to counter the destruction which will otherwise afflict the bleached strands.

Another trend, which resulted from the hippy era of the 1970s, is that many people wanted to try natural hairdyes again, in preference to the chemical ones, and the industry has experienced an enormous boom in henna dyes for darker hair and cammomile—a mild natural bleach — for lighter shades. Henna is also sometimes mixed with metal salts to give non-reddish colours but these additional compounds can unfortunately cause toxic reactions.

HIDING THE GREY HAIRS—METALLIC HAIR DYES

A more recent problem than the general hair dye scare, was brought to light in Australia by the Consumers' Association there, which looked at *Grecian 2000* and the various rival hair dyes on the market designed to counter the ageing effects of greying hair. Contrary to what consumers might think, and the manufacturers' ads promise, these metallic dyes do not restore natural hair colour, but instead add a metallic coating to disguise the grey.

Not surprisingly these anti-greying products are very popular with men as well as women. However, because grey hair looks very similar to the bleached hair, as worn by Linda Evans, many older women at the moment positively encourage their grey hairs because they look fashionable and attractive to many eyes.

According to the ACA researchers, many metallic dyes are poisonous, especially those containing lead acetate, which is both carcinogenic and terato-genic (increases the incidence of foetal abnormality). I took up the criticisms made in Australia, with Combe International, the company which makes and distributes *Grecian 2000* in the UK. They described the report as being 'grossly inaccurate' and insisted that the *Grecian* products were 'among the most thoroughly tested and safest cosmetic products in the world and, accordingly, we have no plans to change the formula.'

They added that only tiny amounts of lead acetate were contained in the *Grecian* products and that since everyone was exposed to lead in the environment, every day the small additional amounts were not hazardous. (This is the same argument, incidentally, that the nuclear industry employs in favour of expanding nuclear power, by arguing that, as we are exposed to background radiation anyway, a little more does us no harm.)

Such reassurances may not satisfy all of us; they certainly do not satisfy me. The fact that we are already exposed to dangerous substances known to be poisonous to humans means we should minimize additional contact, not accept it because we are already exposed anyway.

In defence of its *Grecian* products, the manufacturers insisted that lead acetate could not be absorbed through the skin. It quoted a research study carried out by Dr Abraham Goldberg (who later became chairman of the government's drug safety watchdog, the Committee on Safety of Medicines), which used a sophisticated radioactive isotope trace technique which showed that lead acetate could not be absorbed in this way.

It was upon this research, apparently, that the regulatory bodies approved the use of lead acetate in certain cosmetics products in America. *Grecian 2000* products are sold in America but the latest information is that the safety experts at the Food and Drug Administration are evaluating lead acetate's risk as a possible carcinogen.

DANGERS TO PEOPLE WORKING IN THE INDUSTRY

What about the people who work in the industry that produces all these chemical hair products? Ten different medical studies have shown that cosmetics workers and hairdressers are *ten times more likely to develop cancer than might otherwise be expected*.

Hairdressers and their industry spokesmen refuse to acknowledge any significant cancer risk whatsoever, but when you consider that roughly half of us dye our hair regularly, and that the sector is worth an estimated $280 million a year for permanent dyes alone, you can begin to see why there is a conspiracy of silence.

> 'The attractive scents and packaging used by products in this industry mask potentially serious health hazards.'
> *President of the UFCWIU*

A massive amount of work has been done in America by the United Food and Commercial Workers International Union (UFCWIU) which represents over 500,000 employees of the cosmetics and hairdressing industries.

A recent special report presented to

the US government by the UFCWIU calling for more protection for cosmetics industry workers, stressed the hazards of repeated exposure to a host of toxic chemicals — particularly in hair products.

In a frightening letter to the Government, the union's president William Wynn listed some of the terrifying chemicals used especially in the manufacture of hair products. He pointed out, 'The attractive scents and packaging used by products in this industry mask potentially serious health hazards.'

Some consolation for the public, if not the people who work in the manufacture of the products and the beauty business is that at least products intended for use by consumers at home have to carry warnings if they contain any hazardous chemicals.

Shame on you if you have ever used a perm or hairdye at home and skipped the tedious business of wearing the (albeit flimsy and badly fitting) plastic gloves supplied in the pack! Hair products are among the most chemically active and dangerous available to cosmetics customers — *use them with great care and respect.*

WARNING

- Think very carefully about using any hair dye. Is it worth the risk?
- If you must dye your hair, follow the instructions exactly, wear gloves and keep the dye off your scalp.
- Do not use permanent dyes.
- Avoid products with strong warnings on the label.
- Do not use products containing parapheylene-diamene (This has to be listed on the label).
- Avoid dyeing your hair during pregnancy.
- If you suffer any reaction, report it to the manufacturer and to the Department of Trade.

A SUGGESTION FOR THE HAIRDRESSING INDUSTRY

Although most manufacturers are careful to warn people using cosmetic products containing strong chemicals at home to test them out first on small area of scalp, it is very doubtful if many buyers do, and if you have your hair done professionally in a salon, this pre-testing is practically never done. Nor do you ever know what substances has been put on your scalp.

It should be a routine procedure for a would-be customer wanting to have her hair coloured or permed to have a skin-test a few days ahead. She should also be told precisely what chemicals are being applied to her head. After all, the hairdressers wear rubber gloves! Why should the scalp be less sensitive than the hands — if anything it should be the other way around as the hands are made of much tougher skin!

But perhaps if we knew in advance that our hair or scalp might react badly, or if we read the full list of ingredients we were paying others to apply, we would not keep those appointments.

In my own case, a set of bleached highlights, carried out in a good hair-dressers, triggered a violent allergic reaction which lasted, on and off, for about three years. This caused an unpleasant period of dandruff which was embarass-ing and, at times, extremely itchy and uncomfortable.

DANDRUFF

David George, a professor of pharma-cology and toxicology at the University of Utah, in America, says dandruff is more common than not, and wants the public to realize that dandruff is not a disease and is not, as some dandruff shampoo ads would have us believe, a mild form of psoriasis or seborrhoea. If one has either of these diseases they will show elsewhere on the body and are not confined to the scalp.

He says, 'Dandruff can be defined as a non-inflammatory scalp condition characterized by excessive scaling of scalp tissue. *Most people have dandruff.*'

This continual sloughing off of dead cells is perfectly normal and takes place on the rest of the body too — but we can't usually see it happening anywhere

> 'Dandruff is not disease . . .
> most people have dandruff.'
> *Professor David George*

but on the head. Because these bits of dead tissue on the scalp are fairly large, instead of falling away on the carpet or the pillow, they get trapped in the hair, combining with oil secretions, dust and other particles to form what we know as dandruff.

David George says, 'There is no way to prevent dandruff, but it can be con-trolled, and there are several approaches to decrease its visibility'.

Despite volumes of research all around the world, nobody has yet come up with an explanation of why dandruff is a problem to some people and not to others.

SOME PRACTICAL TIPS TO REDUCE DANDRUFF

Perhaps the most useful treatment for dandruff is regular shampooing of the hair — especially the scalp — with a thorough massage as you go, not just a cursory smearing on of shampoo. More important is the rinsing. Most people do not rinse their hair properly, leaving it either dull or full of bits of detergent which aggravate the scalp and so cause more flaking!

Whilst they will not stop dandruff, special shampoos containing either selenium sulphide or zinc pyrithione should reduce the level of sloughing off that is taking place in most cases. It is worth experimenting with different shampoos to find the one that seems most effective for you. But shampoos, even if they call themselves 'dandruff-controlling' shampoos will not help much if they only contain anti-bacterial or anti-fungal agents, despite their claims to the contrary on the bottle!

Evidence published in the *Journal of Toxicology and Applied Pharmacology* suggest that zinc pyrithione is both fairly effective and safe. It can be found in *Head and Shoulders* and *Revlon ZPII*.

However, selenium sulphide or sulphate is also effective but is potentially dangerous if used on inflamed areas of the skin and if accidentally swallowed. It is to be found in products such as *Selsun* and *Lenium.*

Professor Sam Shuster of the Department of Dermatology at the University of Newcastle upon Tyne says:

> Anti-dandruff shampoos containing either selenium sulphide or zinc pyrithione will offer some relief to suffers. Although a comparative trial has not yet been done, I am personally convinced that some of the newer drugs that will soon be available will be considerably more effective in eliminating dandruff.

He points out that a bad attack of genuine dandruff or a yeast infection commonly affects not only the scalp but also the eyelids, the sides of the nose and cheek, the upper lip and even the chest and top of the back.

Trying to combat a yeast fungal infection with a cosmetic anti-dandruff shampoo containing no powerful agents, and moisturizers which merely temporarily coat the shedding skin is a waste of time and money. Seek medical help and ask your GP or pharmacist about new products.

Although the pharmaceutical companies are very protective of their new developments, (and the opposite once they are able to market them) keep your eyes open for a new 'Brand X' anti-dandruff shampoo still under trial in 1988 and made by a pharmaceutical company called Janssen. According to Professor Shuster, this product really will eliminate dandruff for most sufferers.

My own feeling—perhaps rather cynically—is that it is obviously in the interests of the cosmetics industry for a sizeable proportion of us to keep having dandruff and itchy scalps. After all, the medicated shampoo market is valued at £50 million a year in Britain. Indeed, the medicated and anti-dandruff market constitutes a solid half of all shampoo sales—so there are obviously a lot of dandruff sufferers around.

And the dandruff shampoo manufacturers are not even satisfied by collaring the millions of us dandruff sufferers who delude ourselves that their products are going to cure the problem. The makers of *Head and Shoulders,* the market leader, starting advertising its product in 1986 'for people who don't have dandruff'. That seems almost an admission that if you do, this product won't help you any more than any other.

Perhaps I might add that my own bout of dandruff only subsided when attacked with a powerful scalp ointment prescribed by my doctor.

SHAMPOOS

Shampoos were only really developed in the 1930s. The early shampoos were pretty harsh and yet today's products still contain synthetic detergents which remove the dirt and grease just as effectively as the old-fashioned shampoos — and indeed, as efficiently as the liquid detergent we use for washing up! However, most modern shampoos are effective without being harsh. Some are very mild and can be used every day for people who feel their hair only looks good when it has been washed.

There are so many shampoos on the market it is very hard to know which to choose. Some people stick to a product they like for years at a time while others succumb to the ads and buy each new product that comes out either out of curiosity or because they still haven't found one they like.

In fact the formulation of most shampoos is very similar (they differ chiefly in the strength of the detergent) so you might as well try the cheapest ones until you find one you like. Remember that if you rinse your hair properly, most of the herbs, oils and other advertised frills will be washed off with the lather.

HOW OFTEN DO YOU WASH YOUR HAIR?

Many of us grew up with the beauty-lore, peddled by most magazines, that it was unhealthy to wash your hair more than once a week, and many a greasy-locked school-girl must have battled with her mother and grandmother—and even herself, to avoid this 'rule'.

If you want a rule, you can say that, if your hair is fair and you live in a town, you will need to wash your hair more often than somone who has dark hair and lives in the country. And if it is worn in a style which needs constant flicking back (like a long fringe for example) your fingers will make it greasy fairly quickly. It is true that you can take too much oil out of your hair if you use a powerful shampoo not designed for frequent washing, and while it won't look greasy, it will look dull and lifeless. The trick is finding the happy medium—as always.

A shower-user could try a mild hair-wash, using only a small blob of shampoo, or just wash the fringe if that is the only bit which is greasy. Active or sporty types who sweat a lot will probably find it easier to wash their hair every time they take a bath or shower, and there is nothing wrong with this as long as the shampoo they use is a mild one.

Some shampoo labels contain the scientific-sounding term 'pH balanced', which sounds impressive and must help to sell the products. the 'pH' of a substance indicates the degree of its alkalinity and acidity, and a shampoo that is 'pH balanced' is supposed to weigh up the alkalinity in the detergent against the acid mantle which protects the hair. If this balance is upset, the theory is that the hair becomes dry, lifeless and dull-looking.

Whatever the claims, many people feel that these 'pH balanced' shampoos are no more effective than an ordinary shampoo and the extra spent on them is probably a waste of money, unless you think such products look impressive on your shelf!

SQUEAKY-CLEAN HAIR IS WORTH £150 MILLION A YEAR

We spend over £150 million a year on shampoos in Britain and the market is growing at an estimated 11 per cent a year. Already two-thirds of women, and even more men, wash their hair at least twice a week. Are we too susceptible to those ads of people with gleaming, silky hair? Let there be no doubt that we are pressured into having squeaky-clean hair.

It is common now for the brand-leaders to spend over a million pounds a year promoting their particular product, especially if it is new. For example, Elida spent nearly £3 million on advertising *Timotei,* the fastest-growing 'cosmetic' shampoo of 1986, despite the fact that it had been on the market already for three years. Consumers hardly need to be told it had arrived. Elida also had the second-best seller in the dandruff/medicated market with *All-Clear* and spent £600,000 in 1986 persuading the public that its product was best. Elida also put another million pounds into promoting its *Sunsilk* shampoos, the ads for which have been dominated by pretty blondes for years.

Elida was not alone in spending like this on advertising shampoos; most of the companies do. For example. Alberto Culver spent £2 million promoting their VO5 range and in 1986 it also came up with the idea of grading the depth of hair-washing along the same 'factors one to three' lines as sunscreen SPF formulas.

It is not just the fashion- and label-conscious younger end of the market which requires such competitive marketing. Johnson and Johnson spent over £2 million in 1986 promoting *Empathy,* a shampoo it launched in 1984 especially for women over 40. But no doubt satisfied with the dominance it exerts over the baby market, it did not actively promote its baby shampoo, but mere repackaged it in larger more economical sizes.

CONDITIONERS—DO WE NEED THEM?

Children and people who have left their hair in its natural state don't need to use a conditioner. If you do, then you will discover that choosing a conditioner is just as complicated as choosing a shampoo.

Nowadays, you can not only buy conditioners for dry, greasy or 'normal' hair (what kind of boring people admit to having normal hair these days?) but also conditioners for perm-damaged hair, dye-damaged hair and for hair that is continuously blow-dried!

Just as a moisturizer puts a protective layer on the skin so a conditioner coats the hair shafts to keep in the moisture. The conditioners that claim to be specially prepared for perm-damaged hair also provide a lubricant to replace some of the sebum which the chemicals in the perm have stripped out of it.

Conditioners, just like shampoos, can be mild and merely make the hair feel silkier and less tangled, or they can be rich and nourishing, which can make the hair feel so heavy and greasy that it needs another wash! The rich conditioners usually have to be applied to towel-dried hair and then wrapped in a warm towel for at least 20 minutes. This is equivalent to putting a rich moisturizer on and sitting in a steaming bath.

Greasy hair does not need a conditioner except on rare occasions such as after prolonged exposure to sun and sea. If your hair is really dry and out of condition, you can either buy a deeper oil-based treatment, or a henna-wax product, or use plain old cooking oil from the kitchen (olive oil is supposed to be good). I find that all these oils, including the commercial ones, stick to the hair like glue and the only way you can get them off immediately is by using a liquid detergent designed for dishes—which rather defeats the whole point. Ordinary shampoos just don't have the 'muscle' these days to shift that kind of grease and therefore if you feel your hair needs the oil treatment, you will have to put up with greasy hair until you've washed it several times.

HAIR REPAIR PROTECTION

The cosmetics industry recognizes that many of its products can cause serious damage to your hair and some of them make special shampoos and other hair products to try and repair it to some extent. For example, Estée Lauder has recently launched a *7-Day Repair Complex*, which costs a hefty £27.

CHAPTER FOURTEEN

PERFUME

WHO WEARS PERFUME AND WHY?

Most of us wear perfume, as we wear all other cosmetic, toiletries, clothes and hairstyles, to enhance our attractiveness to our associates and to the opposite sex.

In a survey carried out by *She* magazine in 1985, 95 per cent of readers said they wore perfume and between a half and a third wore it every day. Interestingly, more than three-quarters reckoned that perfume was a necessity rather than a luxury—only one in twenty rated the wearing of fragrance as a treat.

To show how much we now take perfume for granted, another survey carried out by MORI found that women preferred, by three to two, a box of chocolates to perfume and, by four to one, they voted for breakfast in bed in Valentine Day, in preference to a bottle of perfume!

In the *She* survey on perfume, men were also asked their views and habits and three-quarters said they used aftershave, whilst 37 per cent used a cologne or perfume. More than a third reckoned fragrance enhanced their attractiveness to women, whilst 10 per cent said it gave them more confidence at work. Interestingly, only 7 per cent of men bought their own fragrance whereas many women bought perfume for themselves.

COMPANY PERFUME

One employer insists that all his female staff wear his favourite scent—at £50 per bottle. He says the £300 per month it costs him is worth it to stop the 'clash of odours'.

It is clear that we rate the way we smell very highly, as in Britain we spend well over £400 million a year on about 50 million bottles of perfume. There are between 250 and 300 scents to choose from on sale in the shops at any one time. Most sales are of scents for women, although about a third of the total expenditure now goes on men's colognes and aftershaves. Furthermore, the fragrance market increases at the rate of about 16 per cent each year, which is an enviable growth-rate for any kind of industry.

Worldwide, we spend a staggering $2 billion on fragrances of all kinds, which perhaps explains why there are so many new perfumes always being launched.

In Britain, the most popular house is Estée Lauder, followed by Yves St Laur-ent, Chanel, Dior and Parim, and we spend nearly £300 million on these prestige brands. We spend another £100 million plus on the mass market brands, of which Lentheric, Morny and Yardley (all part of Beechams), are the best sellers, followed by Avon, Coty, Revlon and Max Factor.

> Madame Pompadour is said to have spent £40,000 per year on perfume. A fair outlay for the 18th century.

WHOSE NAME ON THE BOTTLE?

We find the designer names attractive, but in fact few of the famous names attached to the bottles appear to have anything to do with the actual selection of the scent marketed under their name, and even less to do with the production of it, aside from the original promotion and photo-call.

Liz Taylor did, however, make a point of saying specifically how much she was going to be involved with the perfume that she has endorsed. Before Parfums International embarked on its $10 million launch of *Passion*, Miss Taylor in-sisted she was 100 per cent behind the product:

I've blended my own perfume for years, and this was as close as I could get. We called it *Passion* because someone once asked me what I thought was the ingredient within me which made me what I am and I said I thought it was my sense of passion.

At about the same time, ballet dancer Mikhail Baryshnikov was also said to be lending his name and image to a new perfume but, somewhat diplomatically, it was apparently made a condition of the marketing tactics that the perfume bearing his name would never be sold in Russia, the country from which he had earlier defected.

'Designer' perfumes invariably belong to major industrial groups, for example *Poison* and *Dioressence* belong to the champagne firm Moet Hennessy, while *Givenchy* belongs to the Louis Vuitton luggage firm. Similarly *Femme* and all the Rochas perfumes belong, along with Balanciaga, to the German drug company Hoechst.

Designers like Ralph Lauren, Yves St Laurent, Gloria Vanderbilt and Emmanuel Ungaro are usually paid commission on sales of the perfumes which bear their name and image, and this money often subsidises their work in the expensive fashion world. Almost 68 per cent of St Laurent's sales are accounted for by royalties, whilst at Dior it is 30 per cent and at Chanel it is a mere 3 per cent.

Many of us make the mistake of choosing scent because we like the ads, or the bottle. This is not so daft considering the bottle and the packaging are invariably more costly than the perfume!

Some packaging is pricer than others. For example, *L'Air d'Or,* which sold exclusively in Harrods for £8,000 a bottle, contained flakes of 23 carat gold. Then there was *Iamyne,* which cost £1,230, including the real diamonds in the stopper, or *Le Parfume Salvador Dali,* which, at £2,400 a time, means that the few bottles sold will probably become valuable antiques one day! Chopard's *Happy Diamonds* perfume was launched in 1987 with more fanfare for the exquisite diamonds and jewellery than for the scent itself. But affluent customers got a 'free' diamond set in 18 carat gold, which was released in the bottle when the last drop was used.

FINDING THE RIGHT 'PONG'

Regardless of how cheap or expensive the scent, the worst thing we do is to overdo the application so that the scent is overpowering and quite unpleasant. Napoleon must have had a pretty overwhelming odour considering he is reputed to have doused himself in a whole bottle of the scent made especially for him, every day! The Japanese, who use little perfume, or deodorant, invented the air-freshener specifically to fumigate their homes after 'smelly' westerners had left.

Most people by now know that perfume smells very different on the skin from how it seems in the bottle, and also smells different on each person as individual skin chemistry reacts with the perfume. It is, therefore, vital to test perfumes before buying. Most new fragrances offer trial samples and it is always worth asking sales assistants if you can have one. The professionals' advice, incidentally, is to never try more than three different perfumes at a time otherwise your nose cannot distinguish the separate smells as they settle on the skin. Your sense of smell also changes throughout the day, and is altered by strong food, such as curry. Research by the *National Geographical* magazine suggests that factory workers have a stronger sense of smell than outdoor workers.

Musky perfumes must smell good on some people otherwise they would not sell in the numbers they do, and the art of choosing perfumes is in knowing what smells good on us to others, not merely to ourselves. Estée Lauder's *Cinnabar* always attracts positive comments from other people when I wear it, yet I think it is pretty obnoxious when first applied. And, whilst my personal favourite is Chanel's *Crystalle*, I've yet to receive any compliments when I am wearing it!

Generally speaking, we wear perfume to make us feel pampered, sexy, pretty powerful, classy, or whatever is our particular mood at the time. Some wear perfume constantly, whilst others use it either when they feel 'special' or simply when they remember to put it on.

Whereas women used to have one favourite fragrance and stick loyally to it, the mass market has ensured that these days most men and women wear a variety of different scents, according to mood, the occasion and what they wear and intend to do. Self-purchasing is on the increase, although still about half of all perfume is bought for gifts.

Although some perfumiers deliberately set out to overpower (as Calvin Klein did when he devised *Obsession*), most of us actually dislike the smell of strong perfume, almost as much as the smell of rancid body odour.

This is true whether at work or play and on men or women. A man who reeks of aftershave, whether expensive or cheap, is as unattractive to most women (and other men) as the women who smell as if they have accidentally tipped the bottle on themselves.

THE PSYCHOLOGY OF PERFUME

At a conference in England in the summer of 1986, psychologists from various parts of the world got together for the first time to study the psychology of perfume and how it could be usefully applied beyond cosmetic purposes. It has already been found that certain types of smell arouse certain emotional rections in people. Dr George Dodd of Warwick University, where the conference was held, reckons it will not be long before perfumiers are designing fragrances deliberately to evoke some particular emotion from those in close proximity to the wearer.

Medically, the smell of peaches and plums seems to bring relief to backache sufferers whilst there is the possibility of certain scents being used to treat depression.

Already, scientists have found that the strong smell of apples, especially when combined with spice, has a relaxing effect and reduces stress in some people, even lowering their blood pressure. In America, perfumiers are working on 'alertness' fragrances consisting of mint, pine and eucalyptus, which are designed to make people perk up at otherwise soporific meetings.

Have you ever noticed how a particular smell brings back some memory of childhood say, or an ex-lover, or a particular house, or type of activity? Well, the perfume industry is now looking into developing scents that will stimulate failing memories, so that elderly people, or people with poor memories, could squirt a bottle of 'eau de dusty volume' or 'eau de log-fire', for example, to revive some deeply buried memory or events otherwise lost to them.

Human olfactory powers are very sensitive and powerful indeed. However, evolution has led to humans abandoning the art of smelling, relying more on the eyes and ears for communication. But this instinct is not lost, for a one-month-old newborn baby can sniff out its mother's clothing from a pile of newly washed garments, even distinguishing hers from other breast-feeding mothers' clothes.

Most of us do respond positively and warmly towards someone who smells good. Few are lucky enough to have such an aroma that is 100 per cent natural. Wearing clothes which smell fresh and delicately perfumed can be more attractive than wearing a clearly identifiable perfume along with smokey clothes with a lingering odour of stale sweat.

It is said that in the sixteenth century, the Duke of Aragon fell madly in love with Marie of Cleves, not because she was a beautiful 16-year-old, but because after dancing with him, she became sweaty and withdrew to change in a nearby dressing room. Afterwards, the Duke, mistaking the room for a cloakroom, inadvertently wiped his brow with her discarded blouse and from that moment on, became passionately attached to her, magnetized by her sweat!

PERFUME AND AGGRESSION

Research highlighted by David Lewis in *Loving and Loathing: The Enigma of Personal Attraction,* has shown that men respond more aggressively towards women who wear perfume than those who do not. However, the style of dress is an important factor, for dressed-up ladies wearing perfume seem to have an off-putting effect on men, but, when presented with women wearing casual clothes, perfume has the effect of making the wearer appear warmer and more appealing. What this research, carried out in America, showed overall, is that women who wear perfume risk arousing aggression.

Think about that, next time you put on your scent before setting out on a dark night. Or as David Lewis asks, 'Are people who spend a fortune perfuming themselves in the hope of adding to their appeal simply wasting their time and money?'

WHY DOES PERFUME COST SO MUCH?

In a bottle of scent costing anything from £10 to £60, the actual ingredients may only cost a few pence, but what we pay for is the research, the packaging, the design of the bottle, the image, the ads, the marketing, the lavish launches and all the hype that goes into making a new scent a successful seller. Every year, about 50 new fragrances are launched and some, like Cacherel's *Anais Anais* and Chanel's *Coco,* go on to become 'classics', whilst others, like *Fergie* and *Sophia,* quietly disappear after a brief moment of fame.

Before *Poison* was launched, for example, Christian Dior spent a staggering £10 million getting all the essential 'extra' ingredients right. Yet the investment has clearly paid off, with the initial costs already just about recovered, and the future set to bring at least £2–£3 million a year from this one scent alone.

When Dior launched *Poison,* they held a 'small' party at The Hippodrome costing £250,000; for the launch of Chanel's *Coco,* Le Gavroche, the ultra-expensive French restaurant, was hired; and Oscar de La Renta took a large party to the Royal Ballet to announce the arrival of *Ruffles*.

Other perfume companies throw in free five-star foreign trips to sumptuous places—Krizia for example, took a party of British journalists to his palace in Milan to launch *Teatro Alla Scala,* the perfume named after the famous opera house, while *Fendi* was launched amid an audience of international celebrities at a gala in Rome.

It is not just women's fragrances that are launched in such extravagant sytle. L'Oreal invited the same fortunate group of beauty journalists to Paris for the launch of Ralph Lauren's *Polo* and Yves St Laurent went one better by flying them to Paris, and also by persuading Rudolph Nureyev to dance at the launch of *Kouros*. Karl Lagerfeld took over the palace of Versailles and laid on a glittering party which cost £500,000 for the food and champagne alone when he launched his *KL for Men*. Back home, Hever Castle was used as a scenic backdrop to launch Estée Lauder's new *Tuscany* and L'Oréal had a champagne breakfast at the new London Tiffany's to launch *Paloma Picasso*.

And so the sumptuous merry-go-round of lavish parties continues. What all these launches aim to do is get their perfume talked about, sought after and considered desirable by as many people as possible. A really successful fragrance will easily rake in millions of pounds a year if it hits the big league. Worldwide sales of *Chanel No 5,* for example, are said to top $50 million every year, and already the sister perfume *Coco* is said to be making two-thirds this sum.

PERFUME: SOME TECHNICAL FACTS

When you open a bottle of perfume, the first smell is the 'top note', which is the most volatile element of the product. After about five to twenty minutes, the 'heart' of the perfume can be smelt and this is the 'body' which will smell different on different people. If you still feel overpowered by a perfume after 10 minutes, then it is too strong for you. The scent should last for between two to four hours on the average person.

Incidentally, smoking interferes with the body's chemistry and will affect any perfume you wear. People who give up smoking often find they have to change to a lighter fragrance not only because their sense of smell becomes more sensitive, but also because others can smell their perfume better without the tobacco smoke. Similarly, some types of medicines can interfere with perfume, especially anti-depressants which can decrease the amount you sweat. Hot climates can also affect the chemicals in your skin by making you sweat more, produce more salt and change the perfume you usually wear.

The industry has a vast choice of scents, with more than 200 essential oils, or natural fragrances, added to which there are another 3,000 fragrance compounds which are either synthetically produced or derivatives of natural perfumes.

The perfumiers add various ingredients to 'fix' the scent and extend the 'body' of the product, and these include balsam Peru, balsam tolu storax, benzoin coumarin and, more rarely these days, musk.

Some of the ingredients are not very appealing, especially those in the most expensive perfumes which often contain precious animal proucts—such as ambergris from whales, musk from deer, civet from cats and castoreum from beavers. Perversely, the cheaper scents are more likely to use synthetic substitutes which may be more acceptable to most users. (See chapter six.)

A typical perfume contains up to 20 per cent of the perfume compound itself, but usually much less, with 70 to 90 per cent alcohol and between 4 and 30 per cent water. The perfume compound is both too expensive and too concentrated in its undiluted form. The less concentrated toilet waters, colognes and eau de perfumes are, therefore, generally more affordable and popular. There are no legally-defined minimum concentrations for these and some compounds can be too weak to smell on the skins of some people for more than a passing moment. Colognes generally contain 2–5 per cent of perfume and toilet waters are a little stronger with 5–8 per cent concentration. If you use colognes, you should get into the habit of topping up throughout the day or evening if you want to continue smelling good.

A good 'cheat', by the way, is to use your favourite fragrance in its bath-oil form, rubbed directly on to the skin after a bath when the pores are open. This seems to last longer than the cologne version in most ranges. If you use the fragrance in all its forms: soap, talc, etc., as well as scent, this emphasizes the smell which then lingers pleasantly all day as the different 'layers' wear off.

These days, perfume is not merely sold on its own, but is a vital ingredient of a vast array of cosmetics and toiletries. As such, it is often the key 'creative' component in a product, which may be remarkably similar to all its rivals, except in its scent. Toiletries such a bubble baths, bath-oils and bath salts commonly contain only about one per cent perfume and often much less. This is also true of hand-lotions and body-creams, talcum powders, hairsprays, shampoos and deodorants. This tiny percentage of perfume makes the enormous prices charged for the 'match-ing' products in expensive perfume lines particularly outrageous.

PERFUME PROBLEMS

Perfumes are generally considered to be the main sensitizers in cosmetics so that if a rash or other allergy materializes, the perfume is normally the first suspect. Balsom Peru, for example, causes many people to have an allergic reaction and may be present in several different perfumes. This means that patch testing on your skin is essential, not just to experience the 'body' of the perfume rather than the topnote, but also to determine the perfume is likely to provoke an allergic reaction.

Some perfumes are also photosensitive so that, when worn in the sunlight, they are no only irritating but can also cause brown patches on the skin. Substances known to cause trouble in sensitive individuals include bergamot, lavender, cedar wood, neroli and petrigrain.

Some perfumes which do not cause problems when they are fresh, can become problematic to the wearer as they age in the bottle. This can also happen in reverse, which is very confusing and suggests that it is perhaps worth hanging on to a favourite perfume that causes irritation initially, as it may become more comfortable to wear as it ages in the bottle.

FAKE PERFUMES

A feature of many London streets, especially outside the department stores in Knightsbridge and Oxford Street, are the men who sell the counterfeit bottles of expensive perfume for a fraction of the real price. Convincing as these may seem at first, they usually contain the words 'copy fragrance' in small print somewhere on the packaging. The bottles are also often a different shape from the real thing.

The industry understandably gets very angry with these con-merchants and there have been several successful prosecutions recently. One gang in particular would have made £2 million from sales of fake bottles of *Joy* (the world's most expensive perfume), and *Miss Dior* if they had sold the stock they had. When they were caught, a quarter of a million bottles had been manufactured and were ready for filling with the fake perfume and selling on the streets. Occasionally, these fakes have even been sold in shops, and from time to time chemists' shops are prosecuted for selling counterfeit goods, unlike the street-deals, at about the same price as the real thing.

Although these fake perfumes may seem to be a bargain, they are in fact a waste of money because although the initial 'top note' smells convincingly like the real thing, echoed by the imitation packaging, the effect wears off rapidly and then smells either of nothing at all, or something rather nasty.

BEST SELLERS

From time to time, the cosmetics industry produces lists to show which are the best-selling perfumes of the time. The most recent of these published by Syndicated Data Consultants (in 1986) showed the following results:

WOMEN'S

(All fragrances)

1 *Opium.*
2 *White Linen.*
3 *Youth Dew.*
4 *Chanel No 5.*
5 *Anaïs Anaïs.*
6 *Cinnabar.*
7 *Rive Gauche.*
8 *L'Aimant.*
9 *Charlie.*
10 *Panache.*

It was curious that neither *Fidji*, which has been very popular for years, nor *Coco, Poison* nor *Giorgio* rated in this top ten, but perhaps if a similar survey were carried out today, the list would feature these fragrances.

Taking mass market fragrances alone, the popularity stakes went as follows:

1 *L'Aimant.*
2 *Charlie.*
3 *Panache.*
4 *Tweed.*
5 *Cachet.*

MEN'S

Of the men's range of fragrances, the list was:

1 *Aramis.*
2 *Brut.*
3 *Old Spice.*
4 *Paco Rabanne.*
5 *Mandate.*
6 *Kouros.*
7 *Blue Stratos.*
8 *Givenchy Gentleman.*
9 *Denim.*
10 *Eau Sauvage.*

THE PERFUME FAMILIES

Although there are thousands of different possible ingredients which can be and are used in perfumes, broadly speaking, they can be classified into four basic types: florals, citruses, chypre (woody) and oriental.

There is also a fascinating genealogy of perfumes which charts how 'families' of scents develop from one another down the 'generations'. *Charlie* (1972) for example, is 'descended' from *Fidji* (1966) and *Diorissimo* (1956) on the one side, and from *L'Air du Temps* (1948) and *Joy* (1935) on the other. Similarly, Revlon's *Intimate* (1955) is a direct 'descendent' of *Miss Dior* (1947) and a cousin of *Femme* (1942), *Cabochard* (1958) and *Ma Griffe* (1944). *Intimate*'s 'descendents' include *Cachet* (1970), *Forever Krystle* (1984) and *Ysatis* (1984).

Of the orientals, *Opium* (1977) is a direct descendent of *Youth Dew* (1952) whilst *Obsession* (1985) is descended from *Must de Cartier* (1981), *Chantilly* (1941) and, way back in 1925, from *Shalimar*.

What is interesting about studying the genealogy of perfumes is that you realize that although you have chosen fragrances you like apparently at random over the years, in fact you have probably been drawn to the same related scents. For example, if your favourite fragrance is *Anais Anais*, you probably also like *Lauren*, *Fidji*, *Diorella* and *Muguet des Bois* and if you like *Chanel No 5*, you probably also like *Arpège*, *Je Reviens*, *L'Aimant* and *Madame Rochas*.

THE MAIN PERFUME GROUPS

FLORALS

These scents are very popular with both older people and young girls, being fresh, youthful and light. These were the earliest fragrances because they were based on widely available and easily grown flowers, like lavender and jasmine. Early perfumiers, and amateurs, would crush the petals from these highly-scented flowers and others such as roses, violets, lily of the valley and hyacinths.

Examples: *Arpège, Blue Grass, Beautiful, Calèche, Chanel No 5, Chloe, Coco, Diorissimo, Estée, Fleur de Fleurs, Joy, Giorgio, L'Air du Temps, Le Jardin, Paloma Picasso, Vanderbilt.*

CITRUSES

These are 'outdoorsy' and suit the more athletic sporty types who want to smell like and be reminded of fresh air when they wear a perfume.

Examples: *Anaïs Anaïs, Cachet, Charlie, Eau Fraiche* from Elizabeth Arden, *Fidji, O de Lâncome, Limes* from Floris, *Miss Dior* and *Vent Vert*.

WOODY

These are perfumes based on the smells of the forest—mosses, ferns, sandalwood and woods generally. They are also popular with 'outdoorsy' people who favour a more natural smell of the woodlands.

Examples: *Alliage, Cabochard, Charlie, Chanel No 19, Diorella, Femme, Diva* from Ungaro, *Ma Griffe, Miss Dior, Private Collection, Ysatis*.

ORIENTALS

These are the more powerful heady scents, favoured by people who want to make an impact on others with rich, heavy and sensual, even aphrodisiac aromas.

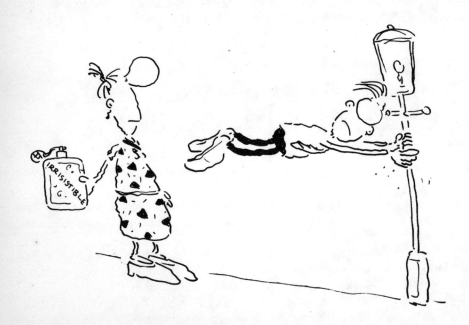

Examples: *Ciao, Cinnabar, Coco, Dioressence, Havoc, Obsession, Opium, Poison, Shalimar, Shocking, Ultima II, Youth Dew.*

Just to be confusing, many perfumes combine some of the above, particularly the florals and citruses, as with Cacharel's *Anaïs Anaïs,* Oscar de la Renta's *Ruffles* and *Parfumes Rare* by Parfums Jacomo.

MEN'S SCENTS

Men's fragrances tend to be citruses and woody smells, rather than florals, although the latter are used in blending. Sandalwood, musk and mossy smells are found in many aftershave and colognes. Leather and tobacco odours are also often included in men's fragrances, but almost never in women's.

Among the most popular spicy/citrus-based scents are *Aramis,* Chanel's *Gentlemen,* Dior's *Eau Sauvage, Drakkar Noir* by Guy Laroche, Dunhill's *Edition,* and *Versace L'Homme.*

Woody smells are found in *Equipage* (also herbs and tobacco), Chanel's *Antaeus, Karl Lagerfeld, Monsieur Lanvin, Macassar, Next for Men, Tuscany, Van Cleef and Arpels for Men.*

Oriental smells are found in *Givenchy for Men, Entrepreneur* and *Old Spice.* Musky smells are found in a wide range of male fragrances which usually bear the 'musk' label.

CHAPTER FIFTEEN
MEN AND MAKE-UP

Men have worn cosmetics and used perfumes and toiletries throughout the ages, and although for the last 150 years or so the fashion has largely been against the obvious use of male cosmetics, there has been renewed interest in 'grooming kits' in the last 20 years. There is now a substantial market for shaving creams, colognes, aftershaves, soaps and deodorants. Currently, the male cosmetics and toiletries market is estimated to be worth about £140 million per year in sales and is growing fast.

Perhaps the most popular male cosmetic aids have been those devoted to the restoration of thinning hair and the colouring of greying strands (i.e. products designed to hide the signs of ageing). More than £1,000 million is spent worldwide each year on various treatments to prevent baldness, so I'll look at that vast section of the market more closely later in this chapter.

Until the 1980s male cosmetics and toiletries in Britain tended to be confined to what men put on their chins and under their arms. However, once 'after-shave'—a clever, functional-sounding name—became acceptable, it was a short step further to persuade men to wear cologne, and an even shorter step to suggest that talc, with its useful drying action, could be comforting, without being effeminate. And now there are signs that the mood among ordinary men is changing and that more cosmetics are coming back.

CATERING FOR THE NEW MARKET

The hugely successful *Body Shop* has recently introduced cosmetics for men, with the emphasis very much on skin and hair care and care has been taken to see that the atmosphere of the shops is not off-puting for male customers.

Among the more up-market brands, Estée Lauder's *Clinique* has a special skin care range for men and several other exclusive names such as Dunhill, Paco Rabanne and Ralph Lauren have jumped on the male moisturizer/ skin care bandwagon.

The UK male skin care market has increased by nearly 70 per cent with an annual spending of around £6 million, of which at least half is spent on the more expensive brands. Indeed when Clinique launched their range of a dozen *'Skin Supplies for Men'*, their spokesman said they had done so because they were aware of a substantial number of 'closet (cosmetics) users'.

Most men still feel awkward about openly buying cosmetics as such, but will happily buy scientific, medicinal, results-orientated creams to protect their skin and lips when skiing, suntanning, windsurfing, sailing or other masculine outdoor sports, whilst 'borrowing' supplies from their wives, girlfriends or sisters for the other things they need. There are also 'unisex' brands like *Nivea* which men will use if they feel the need.

WHO'S SPENDING WHAT?

To show how much things have changed, a survey carried out in the early 1980s suggested that man spent on average a paltry £1 a year on cosmetics and toiletries, and that included shaving creams. Of course, the truth is that women buy these products for their men and, although men say they buy soaps, deodorants, shampoos, conditioners and other hair products, in reality, they use those bought by (and for) the women with whom they live.

However, since that survey was published, there has been a dramatic upturn in the amount of money men spend on various treatments for themselves. A market research survey in 1985 showed that 55 per cent of men said that they were actively involved in the choice of what toiletries they used (even if women actually purchased the products). This tallies with a finding by market researchers in a survey carried out on behalf of Estée Lauder who found that at least 90 per cent of men admitted to 'having problems' with their hair, skin or personal freshness. Perhaps this is why Estée Lauder's *Aramis* range offers a staggering 143 products.

Between 1983 and 1984, there was a 64 per cent increase in the sales of skin care products marketed specifically for men, a 32 per cent increase in fine fragrance brands and a 100 per cent increase in the sales of stick deodorants.

Similar trends have been noted in

other countries. In the last couple of years, French men, for example, have doubled their purchased of toiletries, including shower preparations and bath products, whilst sales of skin care and brilliantines have increased five-or six-fold. In Germany, market research has shown that more than 60 per cent of men's products are actually bought by women, and there is no shortage of brands to choose from. In Japan, hair care products account for three-quarters of the male market, but younger men are reported to be taking more interest in skin care. Despite the fact that oriental men are not very hirsute, shaving products sell extremely well.

The cosmetics industry has not been slow to recognize that the male cosmetics sector of the market was being under-exploited. In 1985 the trade magazine *Soap, Perfumery and Cosmetics* noted that £25 million was being spent by the various companies in advertising and promoting male products. This was £2 million more than all money spent on advertising detergents in 1983. As the magazine said, 'It is clear that a great deal is riding on the new male awareness.'

That figure is a huge under-estimate because it did not include the undisclosed sums spent on advertising by Estée Lauder, whose *Aramis, Aramis 900, Clinique* and other male ranges like *Devin* and *JHL* together account for three-quarters of the male cosmetics market.

Instead of merely selling a one-off bottle of aftershave, to be splashed about on special occasions only, the industry has been aggressively marketing whole ranges designed to get men into using cosmetics and toiletries regularly, like women. While men have been purchasing more of other sorts of toiletries, their consumption of the old standbys of aftershave and talcum powder has actually declined. Perfumes for men no longer have to hide behind the 'after shave label' and even in the up-market brands with designer labels, there are more than two dozen different smells to choose from, and with price-tags reaching the dizzy heights of women's fragrances.

A sizeable proportion of men's aftershave and colognes remain unused on the bathroom shelf, because they have been given these things by women, and men and women have different ideas about what smells masculine and attractive.

MACHO MARKETING

Men's products are always cunningly described. For example *Clinique's* foundation is called 'non-streak bronzer' while the exfoliating cream (which men who shave really don't need), is called 'scruffing lotion'. The 'non-fragranced' hair spray is specifically designed for the man who 'hates or has never used hairspray'. Finally, the spot-concealer stick has the gadgety title 'touch-stick', and its function is to dry up 'skin disturbances'.

Men's skin is made to sound more like the inner workings of the combustion engine, i.e. ravaged components needing 'repairs', whereas women's skin care has traditionally been seductively promoted with a lot of romantic softly worded jargon. (Clinique's PR did point out that the ingredients are identical in men's and women's products—they merely make the men's ingredients 50 per cent stronger. This is probably because men's chins are made of tougher stuff but it makes the men's products much better value.)

The male ranges are not only described in reassuringly manly language and packaged in strong, rugged colours, but they are also directly associated with sport, and sporting events. The marketing of recent new lines has been aimed at the 21 million people who are known to be actively involved in sport in the 1980s health and fitness boom. Look at the number of 'body fitness rubs', otherwise known as colognes and perfumes!

For example, Beecham's managed to make their new *Slazenger Sport* the official deodorant used by the world's leading tennis players at Wimbledon in 1985. The range was designed to appeal to tennis fans and the top end of the toiletries sector of the market, by trading on the high-quality image of *Slazenger*. It is in fact a unisex brand but is sold through sports outlets in a deliberate strategy to reach its target users. Bjorn Borg lent his name and athletic image to a line of Swedish male toiletries launched in 1985.

Another range deliberately exploiting the popularity of current sports enthusiasm is Goya's *Matchroom* which was promoted by leading snooker players Steve Davis, Terry Griffiths and Tony Meo. Thanks to its successful associations with the report Goya announced in 1985 that it was sponsoring British snooker to the tune of £1 million over the next three years on behalf of the *Matchroom* range.

Earlier on, Fabergé's somewhat phallically packaged *Brut 33* was heavily promoted by boxing champions Henry Cooper and Muhammad Ali. (The clever 'macho' marketing of *Brut* in the 1960s and 1970s was perhaps responsible for opening up a whole new market for male fragrance, for the first time making it seem 'butch' rather than effeminate, to 'splash it on'. As *Brut* has a strong musky smell, many women found the effect of all this splashing distinctly overpowering!)

Shulton (the leading mass-market brand, with *Old Spice, Mandate* and *Insignia*) also cashed in on the sports 'aids' market with the *Blue Stratos* sports range. Although sold in chemists, its original promotion included free samples being distributed throughout the nation's sports shops.

Cosmetics companies have also sponsored adventurous activities in an effort to appeal to the macho side of men's personalties. In 1984, French soap manufacturers Roget et Gallet even sponsored a two-man expedition to the South Pole, despite the fact that the intrepid explorers would be unable to bathe more than once a month. One wonders what on earth the team did with the 172 litres of shampoo, 53 kilos of soap, 8 kilos of deodorant and 5.5 kilos of shaving foam with which they were supplied.

A perhaps better-known traveller had his name co-opted to a new men's fragrance in 1985 when Nina Ricci perfumes launched *Phileas,* named after the hero of Jules Verne's novel *Around the World in Eighty Days.* At the same time, Chanel announced sponsorship of the American boardsailing team in association with its new fragrance *Antaeus.*

BASIC SMELLS—DEODORANTS

Sweaty men use deodorants considerably less than 'glowing' women with some 50 – 60 per cent of males claiming to use them regularly, compared with three-quarters of all females. However, market research suggests more men are using deodorants with each successive year and very soon, helped by a lot of aggressive promotion, the industry expects men and women to be equally concerned about body odour.

This is already the case in America where 90 per cent of American women and 80 per cent of American men use deodorants daily, and the industry reckons Britain will catch up in the next couple of years. This is why ever-new male lines contain at least one, if not two deodorants, usually in the most popular form, aerosol, followed by a 'stick' version. Incidentally, the best-selling aerosol brands include *Right Guard, Brut 33,* the combined *Sure* brands, *Old Spice* and *Blue Stratos,* whilst the most popular stick versions are *Old*

Spice, Sure, and *Mennon.*

All of this is particularly interesting because male armpit-sweat has some very significant effects on women... Hidden away in medical journals in the last couple of years have been some fascinating reports about a chemical called alpha androstenol, which is secreted by the male sweat glands under the arms. Research has shown that females are heavily attracted to the stuff, so much so, in fact, that some scientists in the industry have been working on the formula with a view to packaging the stuff and selling it as an irresistible cologne. It would be ironic if men were persuaded to strip themselves of their natural smells, via soaps and deodorants, only to plaster some artificially-concocted version of male armpit sweat on themselves afterwards to appeal to the opposite sex!

The finding has also potential therapeutic benefits, for the University of Pennsylvania School of Medicine has recently found that women's menstrual cycles and fertility can be regularized by thrice weekly doses of male sweat!

We also know that women who live or work together tend to synchronize their periods, but we don't know why. What seems safe to conclude is that body odour may be a very necessary thing for the human race and that overuse of deodorants should perhaps be discouraged. That does not mean body odour should be welcomed back, but regular thorough daily bathing should prevent most people from smelling unpleasant to others. Try telling that to the cosmetics industry though!

NOW MEN HAVE TO LOOK GOOD, TOO

So rapid has the growth in male cosmetics been in the 1980s that in April 1986, *Newsweek* magazine ran a cover feature entitled *You're So Vain—Men Are Primping And Spending Millions to Look Good.* The phenomenon was examined closely and the conclusion reached that males were being forced to look after their appearance in the same way that women have always done, thanks to women's lib.

Noting the large number of New York male executives now patronizing 'beauty' salons (not called that, of course), Michael Solomon, a consumer psychologist at New York University's Business School commented, 'The influx of women into responsible positions in the workplace has shifted the balance of power.' Aside from needing to look good to get ahead at work, these men were also finding themselves having to compete for the attentions of women on a social level. The article commented, 'The vast shift in the dynamics of male/female relations over the last twenty years has had its effects here: men are finding that to attract the women, they need to be, of all things, attractive.'

Other observers believe that the 'shift in the dynamics of the male/female relationship' is a result of the shift in numbers. There have always been more boy babies born than girls, but women used to outnumber men because infant mortality rates were higher among boys. Improved post-natal care has meant that, from about 1960, enough boy babies survived to tip the numbers the other way. Now that men outnumber women, they are having to work harder at making themselves attractive to women—and the explosion of male interest in fashion and cosmetics could well be ascribed to this.

MEN AND THEIR HAIR

Throughout history, it has been acceptable for men to worry about their hair, whether the fashion was for bare chins or whiskers, long curly wigs or brylcreemed slick short-back-and-sides.

Before the advent of constant hot water and ready-made shampoos, merely keeping the hair insect-free and clean was a major job in itself. That was partly why wigs came into fashion and were worn for several centuries from about 1500 onwards. The wearing of wigs by judges and barristers is merely a hangover from the era in which particular wigs indicated your class, income and occupation, as much as clothes and uniforms do today. While aristocrats and courtiers dressed up in flamboyant and elaborate powdered wigs, even the lower social classes of men often wore some sort of wig to enhance their appearance. Wig-wearing died out rapidly after the introduction of a swingeing tax on the use of the accompanying hair powder which in 1795 cost the equivalent of £25 today.

By the 19th century, 'side-whiskers' became the fashion and artificial hair lost its appeal for men, who have only resorted to wigs and hairpieces to disguise hair-loss. The Victorian males favoured whiskers and bearded chins and so did the early Edwardians. During the 1920s and 1930s, men of style imitated the sleek, clean-shaven elegance of people like The Duke of Windsor, Cary Grant and Fred Astaire, and later that of celebrities like Cecil Beaton and Noel Coward.

THE RISE, FALL AND RISE OF BRILLIANTINE

One male cosmetic which has been in use for thousands of years is a hair preparation. Brilliantine—known as bear's grease in earlier decades—was commercialized by Beechams as *Brylcreem*. During the Second World War, the fighter pilots in the RAF became known as the 'Brylcreem boys' and afterwards, in the 1950s, the sleeked-down look was widely copied. So much so, that by 1961, a total of 100 million jars of the stuff had been sold. However, its use rapidly declined in the 1960s and 1970s when shoulder-length flowing locks became fashionable. Then in the 1980s, *Brylcreem* made a comeback, with a re-launch by Beechams, successfully cashing on the neat, groomed look that is once again fashionable with a wide range of people.

STYLE AND COLOUR

Working-class men of little money and less styles, used to dye their greying hair in tea during the 1930s in the desperate struggle to appear younger and to get work. But it was not until the punk era of the late 1970s, that young British men began to style and colour their hair conspicuously. Not everyone has gone in for the long flowing locks of Marilyn and Boy George, nor the outrageous traffic-stopping style of the multi-coloured mohicans who now feature on tourists' postcards, but sunkissed highlights are acceptable these days from the boutique to the City though perms, popular in the 1970s, are perhaps on the wane. Those who do use hair dyes or have perms risk damage to their hair from the chemicals involved. Home perming is especially risky if done inexpertly and if the ammonia is left on the hair too long. Using bleach, which also contains ammonia, can also cause terrible damage. Anyone whose hair starts to fall out after they have dyed or permed their hair should give it a good long rest and wait for the re-growth—and be more careful in future. It may be dead, but it is not indestructible.

HAIR LOSS—A MALE OBSESSION

Men are particularly self-conscious about losing their hair, especially when this process starts when they are young. It is mistakenly considered by them (not women on the whole) as a sign of infertility and failing performance in all things, including sex. Baldness, like grey hairs, also implies advancing years, and this is probably why it upsets so many of the men it afflicts.

> Hair may be dead but it is not indestructible.

Throughout history strange potions have been used to try to reverse the inevitable loss of hair in some middle-aged men, including boar's grease, ground-up parsley seeds, mistletoe, hemp, stinging-nettles, and crushed green walnuts.

These days, doctors and the NHS pay little attention to the natural process of male baldness, and anyone seeking treatment generally has to go to a private clinic. Even Harley Street currently advertises new transplant techniques, but it is impossible to give quotations as these have to be individually analysed. The transplant techniques on the whole have been rejected as frivolous, ineffective or even dangerous by the mainstream medical profession. Anyone contemplating an expensive transplant would be wise to insist on speaking to previous customers, not to rely merely on looking at photographs in a glossy brochure.

> *Hair transplants*
> The medical profession has, on the whole, rejected hair transplant techniques as ineffective or dangerous. Anyone contemplating a hair transplant should insist on speaking to previous customers.

Before we describe the various treatments available, it is necessary to define what we mean by 'hair loss', or alopecia, to give it its proper name.

Normally, hair is lost at the rate of 100 hairs a day or so, and more in spring and autumn, when we moult, just as our pets do. (Don't worry, there are still about 100,000 left on the average head!) Hair loss can be either gradual or sudden—the latter is often temporary whilst the former tends to be chronic with no established medical form of prevention or cure.

TEMPORARY HAIR LOSS

Temporary hair loss can affect both men and women—in women it sometimes occurs after childbirth. Some illnesses, stress, or sudden mental shock or other psychological reasons can trigger a temporary loss of hair. It can also occur as a side-effect of some drugs, especially those used to combat cancer.

IRREVERSIBLE HAIR LOSS

The most common type of baldness suffered by men is called *alopecia androgenetica* and is usually gradual and irreversible. The classic areas for hair loss are the hair line around the face, the hair on the crown of the head and on the pate (the widening parting). In the affected areas, the hairs become thinner and shorter and about a third of the follicles usually eventually disappear.

This kind of alopecia is usually inherited, and often affects men with hairy chests more than those less hirsute. It can be regarded as a sign of masculinity because eunuchs do not go bald, even if there is a family history of male alopecia.

Research so far suggests that the key to understanding and therefore successfully treating male baldness lies in the steroid metabolism. However, there has been excitement recently about the accidental discovery of side effects in some pharmaceutical drugs which apparently offer some restoration of hairgrowth to balding scalps.

MINOXIDIL: A DRUG FOR HYPTERTENSION WITH A MARKETABLE 'SIDE-EFFECT'

For the last couple of years, there has been great enthusiasm because of the discovery that a drug marketed by Upjohn turned out to promote hair growth as well as doing the job it was actually intended to do. (To treat people with such high blood-pressure that their lives were in danger.)

Although the company has yet to obtain universal official approval from the world's drug authorities to market the drug as a hair restorer or cure for baldness, many people, especially in America and Britain, have been obtaining the drug in its present form, grinding up the tablets and applying them to their scalps with some success. Officials in America were very concerned that used improperly, and without adequate pre-trial testing, the drug could cause collapse of the circulation and even death. Thus warnings were issued in the British and American medical press, but needless to say, the unofficial use continued unabated. The drug was even being offered by some hair-restoration clinics on a commerical basis. There was nothing illegal in this, but by using an unapproved drug in this way the operators were leaving themselves open to being sued.

Doctors were torn between wanting to help their patients and fearing being sued if things went horribly wrong. They were also afraid that improper use before the necessary scientific trials had been carried out by the manufacturers could jeopardize the future success of the treatment. Indeed, Upjohn had to threaten legal action against some clinics in America who were taking the treatment too far.

When the formal tests were done, they confirmed the earlier findings and although not every bald head showed regrowth, about 65 per cent did. However, the tests also showed that the hair grew beyond the area of application and that some people suffered skin irritation.

A study published in the *Lancet* in the spring of 1986 suggested that the best results were obtained with younger men with only small bald patches but that with balder men around one third

reported 'good' to 'excellent' results. Results were found to be better if the men wore plastic caps overnight, but these caps gave a significant number of men headaches. (Women are not alone in being prepared to suffer for vanity.)

Canada was the first country to approve *Minoxidil* in a two per cent solution as a treatment for baldness, followed by Belgium. The drug—called *Regain*—is approved by the authorities in America and Britain. It is the first treatment that can truly claim some effectiveness in treating male baldness. Hair loss unfortunately tends to continue when the treatment ceases, and at about £500 for a year's supply, this is definitely something for the affluent only.

THE HELSINKI FORMULA

In the meantime, a non-drug formula, which did not therefore require the approval of the drug authorities, was launched in Britain in 1986.

The *Helsinki Formula* was also discovered as a by-product of a drug, in this case one which was developed by the Finns who were researching into skin cancer at the Helsinki University Hospital.

The product, which costs £25 for a three-month supply, relies on the theory that male baldness is caused by excessive hormone production and it works by using polysorbate and other chemicals to wash away excess male hormones from the scalp area. The treatment involves a shampoo, a conditioner and a vitamin-compound and it is said to reduce hair loss 'dramatically' within two to four weeks. Hair growth is said to follow around three months after beginning the treatment.

When it was launched, the company, Pantron I, confidently predicted that sales would top £3 million a year. In their promotional literature, the manufacturers claimed a 'staggering 80 per cent' reduction in hair loss, and a 70 per cent increase in hair growth in those men who had tried the formula

We are unlikely to be told how many customers took up the company's offer to refund the purchase price if the product failed to give satisfactory results after the first three months!

OTHER DRUGS

A report in the *Lancet* in the autumn of 1986 suggested promising results from research with the drug *Cyclosporin*, which is normally used to prevent the body rejecting donated organs. French dermatologists have found that the drug encourages tufty hair growth and work

is continuing into developing this particular formula as a possible treatment for baldness.

Several other treatments for baldness have been marketed but they have not had the impact on the scientific community of *Regain* or *The Helsinki Formula*.

In 1986, the Australian Consumers' Association investigated a wide range of such treatments, including those offered at specialist clinics, and came to some pretty harsh conclusions:

If you start early enough, there are two ways to prevent baldness; one impossible, the other impractical. You can either choose parents who are not balding and have ancestors who retained their hair into old age, or if you are male, be surgically castrated early in life—eunuchs never go bald. But no matter when you start or how much you pay, there is no way to cure genetically determined baldness. Purveyors of potions and operators of clinics who claim or imply they can prevent, cure or reverse balding should be stopped from doing so—they are taking money from people under false pretences.

A fortune awaits the inventor of the first true *cure* for baldness!

TWO EFFECTIVE WAYS TO AVOID BALDNESS

1 Have ancestors on both sides who kept their hair.

2 Be surgically castrated early in life.

Australian Consumers' Association

Olive oil was reported in 1988 as restoring hair growth to eight bald men in Sweden. Dr Thure Wickhoff made the discovery after recommending a patient with an irritated scalp to rub in olive oil. The man, who had been bald for 50 years, came back with new hair sprouting, as did all the other men who subsequently tried the same thing. It must be worth a try!

SHAVING—GETTING RID OF UNWANTED HAIR

Shaving is the one aspect of grooming common to virtually all men: over 90 per cent shave every single day. It has been calculated that the averagely hairy man will spend 3,350 hours or 19 weeks in front of his mirror, shaving, during his lifetime. Even those with beards and moustaches have to trim round the edges, so there is a vast market in shaving equipment and toiletries currently worth more than £70 million a year.

Aftershave is an item that fills many men's Christmas stockings, and an estimated half of all such products sold in any one year are bought during the Christmas spending spree, mostly by women. No wonder men don't have to buy much for themselves!

Aftershave actually has a purpose—it is not merely for fragrance, but a good product should soothe irritated skin by cooling and even slightly anaesthetizing it, making it feel more comfortable and adding a gentle layer of antiseptic to prevent infection if any cuts have occurred. Unfortunately, and foolishly, most after-shaves are chosen (by women) purely for their smell, which usually accounts for only one per cent of the contents. This is the deliberate intention of the cosmetics industry—which is not concerned about the fact that other ingredients such as witch-hazel, or the alcohol/water balance will have more effect on the consumer's comfort.

There are 16,000 hairs on the average man's face, some of which grow at such speed that fresh stubble appears after only a few hours. This works out at about 800 whiskers per square inch on the chin, and about 250 on the less hairy cheeks.

Whether men shave 'wet', with soap or foam and a manual razor, or dry, electrically, the actual act of shaving sloughs off the top layers of skin. Although if done in haste this can lead to cuts and abrasions, the advantage is that the repeated sloughing of old dead cells, along with the night's hair growth means that men's facial skin is generally in good condition.

It is a matter of choice whether a man shaves wet or dry. Dry shaving is often quicker and less messy, but does not give such a close shave as wet shaving and so is less suitable for darker-haired men or men whose beards grow fast. The combination of water and soap lather removes the oil and softens hair and makes it easier to cut close. The introduction of the convenient disposable razors has probably persuaded many men who previously switched from wet shaving to to dry shaving, to switch back to wet.

Ever since they were introduced nearly forty years ago, aerosol shaving foams have been a popular shaving aid, and are now used by about three-quarters of the male population.

> Save the ozone layer—don't use aerosols.

For electric shavers, pre-shaving liquids help to prepare the skin for shaving by again stripping the hair of natural oils and making it stand erect and thus making it easier to cut. They contain a lot of alcohol and varying degrees of oil so that they help to make it easy to shave comfortably even in warm, humid conditions. Products containing more oil claim to lengthen the life of the cutting blades of electric razors by lubricating them at the same time. There are not many brands of pre-electric formulas to choose from on sale in Britain, presumably because the industry has found there is little demand for them.

RAZOR BUMPS

Men with naturally curly hair often suffer from razor bumps, caused by the hair growing out and then back into the skin. Shaving aggravates the problem by constantly creating little stumps of hair

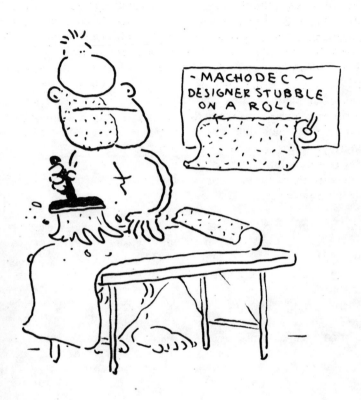

which do this more readily than longer softer strands would. Men who have such hair would be better off giving up the idea of shaving and growing a beard.

Men who are either clumsy shavers or who insist on shaving very curly hair may find a styptic pencil useful in helping their abrasions to heal more quickly.

'DESIGNER STUBBLE'

In the old days, actors who apeared conspicuously unshaved, as Humphrey Bogart often did, did so only to convey characters who had been through a rough time. Even rebels like James Dean and Marlon Brando always appeared with baby-face cheeks. Clint Eastwood was one of the first movie stars to show us that several days' stubble could enhance rather than reduce a man's sexuality. But again that was only okay in the desert or Wild West.

Suddenly, in 1986, 'designer stubble' became fashionable in some, usually artistic, circles. It looked good on certain types of men with finely chiselled features, but on most ordinary chaps, alas, it merely looks scruffy and unkempt. It seems doubtful that the idea will catch on with the majority of men, although it is now possible to buy electrical shavers which are designed to cut the hair to 'designer stubble' length! an easier way to achieve the same effect is to shave at night as most men will end up with the 'designer stubble' look the following morning.

Men who want to adopt this look should wear clean, smart casual clothes and have their hair fashionably cut, otherwise they will merely look as if they got up in a hurry or were put through the wringer, or kicked out of the house the night before (possibly by a lady who didn't approve of their latest cologne!).

CHAPTER SIXTEEN

HYGIENE, BO, AND BAD BREATH!

DEODORANTS AND ANTI-PERSPIRANTS

The cosmetics and toiletries industry has managed to persuade most of us that deodorants are an essential everyday item. In fact, if people bathe regularly enough, do not suffer from profuse sweating problems and regularly change their clothing, then deodorants are probably unnecessary. However, many of us rush about, don't get time to bathe as frequently as we would like to—especially in hot weather—and have a great fear of smelling offensive to other people.

This fear is justified when you consider the findings of a Gallup survey carried out in 1985 which revealed that more than half the 1,000 people questioned worried about working with a 'smelly' person. Nearly a quarter said a BO problem could put them off a prospective boyfriend or girlfriend; 55 per cent said they had at some time moved away from someone on public transport because they smelt unbearable; and 12 per cent admitted that they knew someone quite close to them who had a problem with BO. Of these last, about a third had consciously avoided that person because of the smell, whilst nearly half had bravely tackled the embarassing subject with them.

On the practical side, excessive sweating can also cause unsightly staining on clothing.

People who sweat profusely may be able to seek help from their doctors, although such a problem may be mainly psychological, caused by, for example, a state of nervousness, or connected with a temporary phase of life (such as a holiday or stay in a very hot and humid climate, or a somewhat longer phase, such as the years of adolescence).

In this case, it is worth experimenting with some of the really powerful anti-perspirants on the market such as

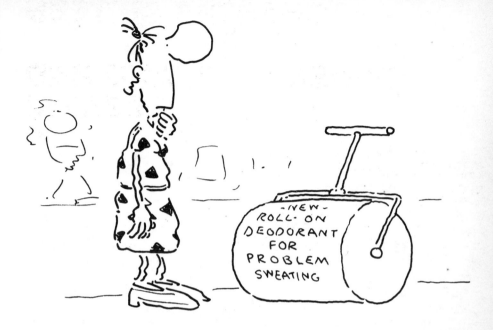

Mitchum, made by Revlon. These really do control 'problem sweating' which can be a nightmare for those affected. Contrary to what you may have heard, there is no evidence that using such a product is dangerous because it blocks the pores. There are plenty of other parts of the body where moisture can escape—and cause less offence and embarrassment!

Having said all that, deodorants and anti-perspirants probably cause many problems—mostly in the form of skin irritations. Out of the ten cosmetic ingredients which have been banned, eight were the main active ingredients in most deodorants and anti-perspirants.

BO is not caused by fresh sweat, but by sweat which has dried and accumulated and become stale. The offensive odour is caused by bacteria breaking down the sweat on the skin, usually under the arms but also between the legs and on the feet. Sweat elsewhere on the body does not tend to smell of anything.

The purpose of a deodorant is to stop the smell by powerful bacteriocides, whilst an anti-perspirant will actually reduce the flow of sweat and kill off the bacteria so that any dampness does not start to smell. Some products have no drying effect and merely prevent odour, whilst others are extremely drying and should be used only by the sweatiest individuals and then not all the time. The most widely-used ingredients are either aluminium salts which reduce perspiration on average by 50 per cent, or zirconium, which usually comes in roll-on form because it has been shown to cause cancer if inhaled.

CHOOSE AEROSOLS CAREFULLY

In 1988, most cosmetics companies bowed to consumer pressure and stopped using fluorocarbons in aerosols.

Friends of the Earth publishes a list of the 'good' and 'bad' products and companies. Companies *not* using fluorocarbons include Nichol and Alberto-Culver. Beecham, Boots, Cussons, Elida Gibbs, Gillette, L'Oreál, Reckitt and Colman, and Schwarzkopf all plan to discontinue them in 1989.

You can contact Friends of the Earth at 337, City Road, London EC1.

AEROSOLS— CONVENIENT-BUT ECOLOGICALLY UNSOUND

Despite the ecologists' fears and warnings about aerosols breaking up the ozone layer which will ultimately lead to a catastrophic warming up of the earth, the public continues to buy the aerosol version of deodorants with about 60 per cent opting for this form, in preference to roll-ons, sticks or creams. Perhaps this is because the sprays tend to dry instantly whereas the roll-ons can remain sticky for some time.

On the safety side, there can be no question that most complaints and accidents occur with the aerosols, either because the spray goes in the eyes, or too much of it is inhaled. (Indeed, some young people do this deliberately and get a 'high' on some kinds of fluids, including one who tragically killed himself doing this in 1986.) So, if the ecological arguments don't convince you, perhaps you will avoid aerosols for reasons of personal safety and use roll-ons. The *American Consumers' Guide to Cosmetics* published by the Science Action Coalition, also recommends that *all* zirconium-based products are avoided, although they admit that the evidence is patchy.

A most tragic accident occurred in

1972 when 39 babies died in France after inhaling excessive amounts of hexachlorphene, which was contained in talcum powder made specifically for babies. The ingredient was a very popular anti-bacterial agent used in deodorants, drugs and some cleaning products. After the babies died and the cause was established, hexachlorophene was banned.

FEMININE HYGIENE PRODUCTS

WARNING

Don't buy vaginal deodorants. If you think you need one, talk to your doctor.

Someone, somewhere, in the early 1960s, decided that the natural fluids secreted by women were so repugnant, both to themselves and others, that it was necessary to introduce vaginal deodorant sprays. For a while, many women rushed out and bought them, and used them every day, convinced that what the advertisers had told them was true.

These days, very few pharmacies bother to stock feminine sprays as so few people use them. What has happened is that women began to realize that they had been conned and even seriously misled. Medical journals began to report the incidence of allergies and irritations to the perfumes and other ingredients in the products and doctors warned women they were not only wasting their money but also possibly risking upsetting the delicate balances in the genital area. Sales tumbled from a peak of $67 million in 1971 to $14 million six years later. This is still, of course, far too much money spent on something that does no good and may do a lot of harm.

For most women, daily bathing is quite sufficient to maintain the genital area in a sweet-smelling state. Possibly during pregnancy, when the hormones make the body slightly sweatier, there may be a need for more frequent bathing, but anyone who feels they need a feminine hygiene product to mask an offensive discharge will amost certainly have an underlying medical condition such as an infection, which will need a doctor's supervision rather than cosmetic disguise. Vaginal secretions are normal and necessary. If you think yours smells offensive, talk to your doctor—*don't* use a vaginal deodorant.

TEETH AND TOOTHPASTE

It's no good having a beautiful or handsome face and bad teeth or smelly breath, or the whole effect will be ruined. 'Manwatcher' Dr Desmond Morris reckons that one possible reason why the Mona Lisa had such an enigmatic smile was because she had had bad teeth! Certainly, in earlier times, it was harder to keep teeth looking white and in good condition.

Whilst women spend £75 million a year on lipsticks, they and the rest of the population spent about £95 million a year on toothpaste.

Dental care is considered so important in America, where everyone aspires to a Farah Fawcett-Majors-type smile, that children are forced to wear braces and get their teeth fixed during adolescence and, as a result, dentists and orthodontists are very rich people. A beautiful set of gleaming even teeth are certainly a very great bonus and a good smile can transform what might otherwise be a rather ordinary face. (Incidentally, smokers and anyone with yellow teeth should avoid red or orange lipsticks which only emphasizes the yellowness.)

Incredibly, half the British population *never* goes to the dentist at all but three times as many women as men attend regularly for check-ups, reckoning quite rightly on the importance of a nice smile. Yet, perversely, lazy as they are about dental hygiene, men are far more ready to point out if a partner has bad breath than women are.

In Britain, since the NHS put the prices of dental care up, dentists have observed that even in more affluent areas, patients are cutting down on their routine visits. Yet teeth are very important—more so even than skin—and neglecting them early on can have dramatic and irreversible effects. There is also a great deal that dentists can do in cosmetic treatments, to improve a bad set of teeth and gums and make a face altogether more attractive, if you are prepared to spend the money.

The dental health products market is worth £125 million in the UK and there is a vast range of toothpastes on the market, each claiming to be better than the next. The aim of all these products is to cleanse, freshen and prevent decay. Colgate Palmolive, Beecham, Elida Gibbs and Proctor and Gamble are the main companies, sharing 85 per cent of the toothpaste market and owning the top ten best-sellers. The companies together spend about £15 million a year trying to persuade us that theirs is the superior brand.

Although there has been a campaign against adding fluoride to drinking water supplies, young children now suffer considerably less tooth decay than their parents did—even though the consumption of sugary food and drinks is higher. This is undoubtedly thanks to the use of fluoride toothpaste which is estimated to reduce the incidence of dental decay by 25 to 30 per cent.

Because the dental authorities are so heavily in favour of the stuff, 95 per cent of toothpastes now contain fluoride and it is quite difficult to buy a toothpaste which doesn't contain fluoride. There are gels, such as *Close-up* which contain corsodyl, which acts as a mouthwash too, but dentists believe gels are no better than fluoride toothpastes.

Whatever toothpaste you use, the product is only effective if you brush well. A cursory wipe with an aged brush over the top of the front teeth will still leave a substantial amount of plaque—which contains bacteria—on the rest, where decay can take place.

Most popular toothpastes contain completely synthetic ingredients—in the old days they used to use chalk. Only about 1 per cent is flavour although researchers say 30 per cent of us choose our toothpaste according to taste.

There is no need to apply as much toothpaste on the brush as the ads suggest—a pea-sized blob is all that is required. However the mouth should *not* be rinsed afterwards, just the excess spat out, with the remaining left on the teeth as a protection.

Brushing without toothpaste is better than nothing, but toothpaste is abrasive and helps shift the kind of bacteria that cling to the teeth in the form of plaque and become destructive. If you dislike the idea and taste of most commercial toothpastes, you can buy herbal formulations from health food shops, containing mint and sage and other natural ingredients.

'Pump' dispensers were introduced in the early 1980s and now about 20 per cent of us use them instead of the old-fashioned tubes which have always been fiddly things and the source of much marital and domestic friction!

About half the population suffers from sensitive teeth at one time or another, often in the form of a painful reaction to cold drinks and food. There are various toothpastes specially designed for such people of which *Sensodyne* is easily the brand leader, thanks mainly to high-profile advertising.

TOOTHBRUSHES

Just as most people never look after their face flannels, so do they rarely consider the state of their toothbrushes. These do wear out, and should be changed as soon as they show signs of wear. We purchase about 55 million toothbrushes a year, suggesting we each change annually, if that.

Ask your dentist for advice on the best type for your teeth. Contoured brushes help you reach the back teeth while concaved-edges help get down to the gums, which are just as important as the teeth themselves.

Professor Aubrey Sheiham of the dental department at the University of London recommends using children's toothbrushes, which have smaller heads and are useful for getting round all the corners. He also recommends nylon, because it washes and keeps its shape better, and is cheaper and quicker-drying than bristles. The brush should be medium hard unless the gums are particularly sore as hard brushes can cause damage and soft brushes are ineffective.

Electric toothbrushes are used by a small percentage of people, and are fine if, for example, they act as an incentive to get children to brush their teeth more often. But on the whole, they are somewhat unnecessary and a gimmick that has never really caught on.

Smokers are often tempted to use *Pearl Drops* or *Eucryl* powders for removing yellow stains from their teeth, but some dentists warn against this type of powder, saying it is too abrasive and can weaken the enamel. According to the British Dental Association stained teeth are better dealt with by the dentist each time you go for a check up, when they will undergo a proper all-round scaling and cleaning. This can be backed up daily brushing with non-corrosive paste.

Also available, and more medicinal than cosmetic, are products designed to prevent the development of tartar, a yellowish mineralized deposit of plaque which clings to the edges of the teeth and gums which has to be removed by a dentist or dental nurse. These products may help keep the teeth clean, but are not a substitute for regular dental care.

Flossing and using wooden dental sticks to loosen plaque and keep the gums healthy are all recommended by the dental profession, as any of us who still do visit our dentists regularly will be aware.

Similarly, mouthwashes, especially those with mild antiseptic or germicidal ingredients cannot do any harm and certainly make the breath taste and smell fresher and they can also reduce and soothe mouth ulcers. There is also evidence that some of these products may work against the build-up of plaque and tartar. We spend over £10 million a year on products like *Listerine* and *Listermint*, which are heavily advertised.

Most people buy mouthwashes in the hope that they will disguise or correct bad breath but unfortunately halitosis may be caused by underlying dental or gum disease, catarrh, sinusitis or even some digestive problem, such as a milk allergy and so the product will have very little impact. Using it may prevent the sufferer from getting to the root cause of the real problem.

Finally, falling in love seems to spur people into cleaning their teeth—when surveyed by a toothpaste company, 90 per cent of single men and women said they clean their teeth. However, five per cent of single men *never* brush their teeth—which possibly explains why they are single. Marriage apparently has a good influence on men as married men go to the dentist more often and take better care of their teeth than those who are single.

CHAPTER SEVENTEEN

PROBLEMS
ARE COSMETICS A HELP
OR A HINDRANCE?

ALLERGIES

At least one in three women who use cosmetics suffers an allergic reaction to *something* in the ingredients. Perfumes are common culprits, as are nail-varnishes, which are responsible for a fifth of all cosmetic reactions.

Many cosmetics contain ingredients which can cause spots and blackheads and other forms of skin irritation such as rashes and sores. Often these reactions occur some distance from where the offending substance was applied and consumers do not always realize what has happened.

Without listing all the possible culprits by their chemical names, the most obvious ones which can trigger an attack of acne include the following:

1 The chlorinated hydrocarbons, contained in paints, varnish, lacquers and various oils.
2 Coaltars and topical corticosteroid therapy, all of which are the basis of treatment for seborrhoea and the treatment of dry, sensitive or flaking skins.
3 Petroleum oil, or Vaseline can also trigger acne in some individuals and this is found in a wide range of cosmetics including lipsticks, hand lotions and rouge-creams.

The following ingredients can produce an outbreak of blackheads:

1 Coal tar.
2 Cocoa butter.
3 Coconut oil.
4 Corn oil.
5 Lanolin.
6 Linseed oil.
7 Olive oil.
8 Peanut oil.
9 Polyethylene glycol (present in many moisturizers.
10 Safflower oil.
11 Sesame oil.
12 Many sun screens.

From the list it will be obvious to many sun-worshippers that there is barely a suntan product on the market which does not contain one, if not several, of these ingredients which can produce an unattractive rash of spots.

Other ingredients can produce an unpleasant stinging sensation which can last up to 15 minutes before subsiding, and these include coal tar along with phenol (carbolic acid used in calamine lotion) and propylene glycol (which is used in shampoos and hair dyes). NB Phenol is the chemical used in chemical face peels (see chapter eighteen).

Dermatologists stress that it is very hard to assess the actual severity and frequency of occurrence of side-effects experienced by users of cosmetics because most consumers who experience a bad reaction merely stop using the product and the symptoms disappear, or do not associate the problem with the product, if the manufacturer changes the compound of, for example, a moisturizer, and introduces an allergen. Few tell the sales assistants or the manufacturers, even fewer tell their doctors or Trading Standards Officers. A tiny proportion end up seeing a dermatologist. Therefore, we have to assume that what we do know about any unpleasant side-effects associated with cosmetics is very much the tip of the iceberg.

Of the reported incidents, we know that there are between three and ten severe experiences per million items of cosmetics sold. Yet there cannot be many people who have not themselves at some time found that a particular mascara, eyeliner, lipstick, cream or shampoo has caused a nasty bout of something or other and the offending item has merely been dumped in the bin—or given to someone else!

AMERICAN STATISTICS

What we do know from the manufacturers' own figures is that the top six 'trouble-makers' include, in descending order, hair colour and bleaches, face creams, eye make-up, deodorants/anti-perspirants (including feminine hygiene products), face make-up and hair conditioners.

Hospital and medical figures are pretty much the same except they include nail cosmetics and soap and indicate fewer problems with hair conditioners and face make-up.

BRITISH STATISTICS

In 1979, the Consumers' Association interviewed 11,062 adults all over Britain of whom 12 per cent said they had experienced an adverse reaction to cosmetics in the preceding year. The top six 'trouble-makers' were as follows: deodorant/anti-perspirant (25 per cent), eye make-up (14 per cent), soap (12 per cent), face cream (7 per cent), perfume (5 per cent), and aftershave (5 per cent).

If you look at face-creams, it is not surprising that they figure quite high on the adverse reactions list simply because there are more than 6,000 different ingredients which can be used to make them. Although the ingredients of the creams have to be tested separately, it is particular combinations which may give rise to problems.

THE IMPORTANCE OF LABELLING

Until 1977, it was not possible to find out exactly what particular ingredient was causing which problem because most cosmetics companies refused to reveal exactly what went into their products.

British cosmetic companies are very reluctant to label their products fully. This is for several reasons. The manufacturers do not want to reveal to the rest of the industry what goes into their products, or to the consumer what high proportions of expensive products are made up of cheap raw materials such as distilled water, alcohol and witch hazel for example. Some of the most heavily advertised brands of mois-

turizers are 90 per cent water. Also the lists are likely to be so long that packaging would have to be re-designed, thus losing product image and identity, or a separate leaflet produced to be inserted into the carton. The cost of this would, obviously, be passed on to the consumer, who may or may not be prepared to pay the increased price.

However, in 1977 it became compulsory in America for cosmetics manufacturers to label their products with a full list of ingredients. Although the rest of the world, including Britain, has been very slow to follow, dermatologists now have a better chance of being able to analyse and assess ingredients since many products are internationally marketed.

In passing, it is worth saying that there is labelling and labelling. Unless the list is clear and states what percentage of which ingredients are contained, then a mere list, especially if only the chemical names are used, is not going to enlighten many customers.

Some ingredients are notorious for causing allergic responses. For example, the hair dye paraphenylene-diamene is such a strong sensitizer that its use has been banned in many countries. This was the substance which was cited as the cause of kidney failure in two Belfast women. British manufacturers still use it but are obliged to mention it on the label somewhere so, if you have had an unfortunate reaction to hair-dye in the past, check the labels.

'HYPO-ALLERGENIC' PRODUCTS

Several companies make a selling-point of the fact that their products are 'hypo-allergenic' and most customers are under the mistaken impression that this means that by using these products they can avoid allergic reactions. Unfortunately, this not the case, for all that such companies often do is to avoid using the most obvious allergens, such as perfume, lanolin and irritant colourings.

Since many cosmetics involve literally dozens of ingredients, it is not exactly dificult to simplify the contents. What is extraordinary is that some of the hypo-allergenic lines are very expensive —yet they use quite cheap ingredients. For example, by taking out perfume they are removing what is often the most expensive ingredient in the formula!

The more expensive brands include *Almay, Clinique* and *RoC*. Companies whose products do not claim to be hypo-allergenic say that many people turn to their products because so called hypo-allergenic brands have brought them out in a rash. This is possibly an unfair jibe since presumably only the most sensitive individuals are likely to seek out an hypo-allergenic brand in the first place.

There are cheaper products for the sensitive allergy-prone skin, such as *Simple Soap* or even baby products, which are so mild even the most sensitive adult can usually use them. There are also many very gentle shampoos on the market, including those designed for 'frequent washing' which are worth trying if you have a sensitive scalp or very dry hair.

Finally, if you prefer to buy a hypo-allergenic brand, and you have no problems, then fine, but be careful to buy in smaller quantities if it makes a virtue of containing no preservatives, as this may mean it has a short shelf-life.

EXCESSIVE HAIR AND ITS REMOVAL

Concern about excessive hair, known as hirsutism or hypertrichosis, is quite common among women. Some become very distressed because it is incorrectly regarded as a masculine trait. (Men, on the other hand, worry about having too *little* hair, especially on their heads, chins and chests!)

Surveys of body hair in women not suffering from disorders causing hirsutism have shown that in fact just over one in four have some facial hair, usually on their upper lips, whilst more than one in three have what they consider to be excess hair on the lower abdomen and just under one in five believe themselves to have excess hair on their breasts, usually around the nipple. Genuine excess hair is thought to be caused by a slight over-activity or reactivity to the male sex hormones, the androgens, which all women produce from puberty onwards and which can be especially active during pregnancy. However, many women, especially those worried about their femininity, think they have too much body hair, especially on the face, when in actual fact they do not. Ask a friend whose judgement you trust for her opinion before you embark on expensive and potentially quite painful 'treatment'. Beauty salons and chemists are unlikely to tell you not to use their service or buy their product.

The business of removing superfluous hair is curiously clumsy and although the cosmetics industry has come up with various formulas and methods, most are based on ancient science and all have their drawbacks. Anyone who can come up with the perfect depilatory, which would remove hair swiftly, painlessly, permanently and without irritating side-effects, would be a multi-billionaire.

As with the opposite problem of hair loss, excessive hair problems, though extremely embarrassing and psychologically disturbing for some sufferers, are not normally something which interest doctors. Women with serious facial hair problems can try appealing to their GPs for help, and there are drugs available which can reduce the hair growth. Unfortunately, some of these can upset the hormones in the body and disrupt periods for example, so they are not suitable for any but the most severe cases.

Most women regard superfluous hair as a purely cosmetic problem to be either tackled by using cosmetics or endured as best they can. Endurance and suffering seem to be a very sad fate.

ELECTROLYSIS

The only way of removing hair permanently is by electrolysis. Even done this way, approximately 15 to 25 per cent of the hair may eventually grow back again.

Electrolysis works by inserting a needle into the base of the hair and using a weak electrical current to permanently destroy the follicle. The process is too slow and expensive for large areas like the legs, underarms and bikini area but it is the preferred method for the face or breasts.

Most women don't like the thoughts of shaving their upper lips (or the idea of hair being there at all). They think, erroneously, that shaving makes the hair grow more quickly and thickly. However, the bristliness of the regrowth is definitely a deterrent.

You can buy electrolysis equipment for use at home but this is not to be recommended. About 99.9 per cent of electrolysis is done in salons where even experienced operators will only do a maximum of 100 hairs at a time. Choose an experienced and trained electrolysist—ideally one who is a member of the British Association of Electrolysists. The 400 to 500 members are allowed to put the initials ABAE or MBAE after their names.

The other simpler methods only get rid of hair till it grows back; a few hours later in the case of shaving, or a few days or weeks later in the case of depilation by chemicals or wax.

SHAVING

This is the quickest, cheapest and easiest method of removing hair and is used by most women for legs and underarms. The secret is use plenty of soap and a sharp razor. Don't apply deodorants to newly-shaved skin. Electric razors are convenient and, if you tend to end up covered in blood after a wet shaving session, you may think the extra initial expense is worthwhile, but there is not significant difference otherwise.

CHEMICAL DEPILATION

These products are meant to destroy superfluous hair and discourage further re-growth, which they only do by continuous applications. They are not supposed to have any irritating effects on the skin to which they are applied, but, in many cases, they do.

It is therefore important not to leave the chemicals on the skin too long, and to follow instructions meticulously, as anything strong enough to dissolve hair can obviously have a powerful effect on your skin.

Early depilatories contained sulphides, which although effective, destroying superfluous hair within five minutes, unfortunately smelt pretty awful and also damaged the skin. Some hair removal products still contain sulphides and these should be avoided. (If the labels don't specify, ask the pharmacist.) The results last for 4-6 weeks and re-growth is not bristly as with shaving.

WAX DEPILATION

Waxing is quite a messy way of removing unwanted hair, also time-consuming and often painful. On the other hand, it usually lasts a long time and when the hair re-grows, it is not stubbly and irritating, as shaved hair is. Wax removers usually contain paraffin, beeswax, resin and petrolatum (Vaseline) in various formulations.

Waxing is best done by someone else as the element of surprise in removal seems to reduce the pain. The wax is applied in a warm state, usually with a spatula, and left to cool on the skin. Once it is set it is tested for adhesion and then ripped away in one swift and usually painful movement, taking the hairs with it. The exposed hair follicles often bleed, and some gentle aftercare is often needed, and in sensitive skins—especially in the bikini area—discomfort can last days. Do not use perfumed talc or soaps until the skin has settled down again. If planning a bikini strip before a holiday, have it done several days before you go away, not the day before or you might resemble a newly and badly plucked chicken!

Although various wax preparations are sold for use at home, and ads claim they are simple to use, they can be very messy and you can end up with patchy results, skin inflammation and large lumps of glue stuck to your underwear for days.

Cold wax-strips, which contain resin and trap hairs rather like old fashioned fly-paper used to ensnare flies, are a little easier to use, though usually more expensive. However, don't worry if you fail miserably using them—either wear more generously-cut swimwear, and put up with the natural growth, or use a salon when absolutely necessary for special occasions like summer holidays.

BLEACHING

Although not a form of hair removal as such, bleaching the hair on the legs, forearms and upper lip can make it considerably less noticeable. This is especially suitable where the hair is dark, but not very thick.

CHAPTER EIGHTEEN

WHEN ALL ELSE FAILS UNDER THE KNIFE— COSMETIC SURGERY

Cosmetics, even the best of them, can only make superficial changes to your appearance. In skilful hands, these can bring about certain transformations, but these last only as long as it takes for the make-up or camouflage to wear off and then nature rears its (perhaps ugly) head once more.

For all sorts of reasons, men and women resort to the scalpel. No one knows how many. For obvious reasons, most people choose to conceal their operations from their closest friends, their doctors, and even their loved ones.

For some people, a successful operation can bring a whole new lease of life —to have what you consider a hideous nose made more 'normal' can be a liberating experience. For others who seek to have their giveaway crow's-feet removed, the hope that youth and all its bounties will return is often disastrously misplaced.

Although you may get the smaller nose, smoother jaw line or larger breasts that you wanted, the emotional and physical side-effects can be huge.

Changes to your face or body will not necessarily make you a more extrovert, attractive or powerful person, and the realization of this—not normally until after the event—can lead to depression.

Physical side-effects include loss of feeling in the area operated upon, long-term bruising, scabbing and scarring. You may get a 'frozen face' after a face-lift, or you may not be able to breast-feed after mammaplasty (breast reduction or enlargement), nor may you be able to breathe comfortably through your nose after rhinoplasty (the nose 'job'). These are not the results of the infamous 'botched jobs' but the expected side-effects of such operations when carried out by competent surgeons.

Obviously, cosmetic surgery is something only the individual concerned can decide about. Besides the money, there is a great deal involved, and much motivation is needed for even the simplest operations to be a success, physically, emotionally, and psychologically.

COSMETIC SURGERY AND THE NATIONAL HEALTH SERVICE

Cosmetic surgery *is* available on the NHS, but in *very* limited amounts, and only for certain problems.

Patients are infinitely more likely to get treated on the NHS for things like burns, breakages and gross deformities rather than for drooping eyelids or saggy breasts.

However, you can still ask to go on a waiting list, especially if you are prepared to wait maybe as much as ten years before you have your operation. For some operations, though, in some areas, there may be no point in even putting your name on a list and if you are considering this route, you should find out about the average waiting time before you put your name down.

The College of Health part of the Consumers' Association, has done some excellent work on hospital waiting-lists and regularly publishes updated information which might be useful, but again, they would not rate inessential surgery such as this very highly.

The theoretical availability of such treatment on the NHS is hampered by the shortage of cosmetic surgeons. In Britain, there are 110 consultants, which works out at about one for every 750,000 members of the public. Most of them work in London, and for the private clinics. In America, by contrast, there is a cosmetic surgeon for every 18,000 potential patients.

Doctor magazine reported in 1987 that the shortage of NHS plastic surgeons was so acute that there were only three plastic surgeons covering the 3.5 million population of the Glasgow health region, and similarly, only four for the 2.5 million people living in South Wales. Even in Scotland, where the waiting lists are supposed to be shorter than the rest of the country, a middle-aged woman with a broken nose was recently told by her doctor, 'It won't be done in your lifetime or mine.' She, like many people needing reconstructive plastic surgery, not just cosmetic surgery, was advised to have the work done privately. Unfortunately, most private health insurance policies do not cover plastic surgery unless you either have a GP prepared to 'bend the rules' or generous provision in the 'small print'.

Anyone embarking on a tattoo ought to be aware of the fact that the same Scottish doctor has quoted 280 years (!) as the waiting time before such an unwanted body decoration could be removed.

GOING PRIVATELY...

Cosmetic surgery is a booming industry all over the world, and thousands of people voluntarily undergo operations in the hope of looking more attractive than nature intended. Most of them are not so ugly that other people would stare at them in the street, but their physical defect is one that cannot easily be disguised by some more temporary method, such as make-up or wigs.

Pick up any newspaper in this country and you can find ads for cosmetic surgery; ring the numbers and the chances are you will be given an 'instant estimate' for a new nose, uplifted bosom or a face lift. Yet while business booms, there is undercurrent of disapproval from the medical profession.

On the medical side, many doctors feel it is quite wrong for cosmetic surgeons to advertise their skills directly to the public, and that a family GP should always be involved in any decision to undergo something as serious as an operation. Through their agencies, many cosmetic surgeons are openly flouting the guidelines set by the profession's disciplinary body, the General Medical Council, which is itself powerless to do anything.

WARNING

Make sure your surgeon is a member of the Royal College of Surgeons and, if possible, also of the British Association of Aesthetic Plastic Surgeons (BAAPS). Be wary of 'surgeons' whose names are followed by unfamiliar initials, and, if in doubt, check them with your GP or the British Medical Association, Tavistock Square, London WC1.

COSMETIC SURGEONS— QUALIFICATIONS

One of the problems and causes of controversy in this field is that there are no formal qualifications for cosmetic surgeons. *Any doctor, or even someone who has no medical qualifications, can call himself a cosmetic surgeon.* Cosmetic surgery attracts doctors from different backgrounds—surgeons in Ear, Nose and Throat being a good example. Some of the leading cosmetic surgeons trained in plastic surgery, and developed their cosmetic techniques on a self-teaching basis.

In a special investigation carried out for the magazine *World Medicine,* in 1980, called 'The Cosmetic Surgery Jungle', writer Robert Eagle said, 'I have heard two accounts, both unattributable, of NHS consultant plastic surgeons being paid sums of up to £30,000 to train registrars for private clinics.'

There are undoubtedly 'cowboys' in the cosmetic surgery industry, who are attracted by the lack of minimum qualifications; the apparent lack of controls by any sort of governing body and of course by the sums to be made from the operations themselves.

Periodically, the GMC will take disciplinary action but it only has jurisdiction over *doctors* and often the complaint is against the clinic or its staff —over which they have no control. Even when cosmetic surgeons are involved themselves, proving a claim of negligence or incompetence against them is very difficult indeed.

On the other hand, unlike most fields of medicine, cosmetic surgery is one area in which reputable practitioners are prepared to give evidence against unscrupulous colleagues, probably because they are often called upon to repair the botched operations perfomed by the 'cowboys', and of course, it's bad for business to have incompetent operators giving the industry a bad name.

WARNING

Check with your GP if you are contemplating cosmetic surgery.

The Medical Defence Association, which insures doctors against malpractice suits, has also said it welcomes information received by reputable cosmetic surgeons to help track down and eliminate the 'cowboys'.

One leading cosmetic surgeon, who like most people I spoke to asked to remain anonymous for fear of recriminations, said:

I've come across some quite disastrous cases. For example, one clinic was run by a doctor who had been running an abortion clinic and he turned to cosmetic surgery because he thought it was more lucrative. Surgeons like me are constantly involved in negligence suits brought against the 'cowboys' by patients. Usually they settle by agreement, but otherwise we go to court and fight. The MDA are quite keen that we should assist in assessing negligence . . . There are other reasons why failures happen which do not necessarily mean the surgeon was unqualified to do the job—he could have operated on the wrong patient for the wrong operation—which is a counselling problem —or he could be inexperienced in that particular operation, or he could simply have had an 'off' day, which happens to everyone. It's more cru-cial of course if it happens to be your face under the scalpel.

> When asked how old a certain society lady looked after her most recent face-lift, Noel Coward remarked 'A very old twelve.'

WOMEN ONLY?

The cosmetic surgeons' patients are mostly women, according to most London plastic surgeons. The most popular operations are ones which make people look younger: facelifts, or versions of them, and nose jobs, or rhinoplasty. A full facelift costs about £2,000, while partial facelift—a 'nip and a tuck'—as it is known in the business, is about half this amount, with the effects substantially less dramatic.

Again, most of the patients seeking facelifts are women, with the average age being 55, although some start trying to turn back the clock at the age of 45. However, more men are now seeking facelifts. They account for 10 per cent of all patients undergoing cosmetic surgery in America and about 2 per cent here in Britain. Men mostly turn to cosmetic surgery for help in fighting baldness and for changing features like ugly noses and chins or protruding ears. Studies in America have shown that men's expectations of cosmetic surgery, especially 'nose jobs' are more unrealistic than women's. Surgeons were warned in a report published in 1987 by the American Medical Association that psychological counselling was essential.

In America, facelifts are so common that an attractive female relative of mine was recently asked, 'Where did you get your nose?' The enquirer, a suntanned Californian, who freely admitted to being on her fourth facelift, couldn't believe my relative's nose was an original and wanted the name of the surgeon so she could order one for herself.

In Britain, we tend to be much more reticent about cosmetic surgery, and women who have undergone some kinds of operation sometimes do not tell even their close friends because they feel somehow ashamed of what they have done. It is certainly not a status symbol in this country, but then, nor is having a 'shrink' or analyst.

In other cultures, cosmetic surgery is more acceptable as a form of self-improvement. In Japan, for instance, where competition for jobs is very intense, students who qualify in their chosen subjects often go off and get their noses, ears, chins, or whatever fixed by a cosmetic surgeon before they embark on a round of job interviews.

In a study reported by David Lewis in his book *Loving and Loathing: The Enigma of Personal Attraction* (Constable, 1985), the administrators of one specialist hospital in Japan said that 5,000 students had undergone cosmetic surgery in 1982, and the figures have since increased. In 1972, students accounted for only 15 per cent of the total number of such patients, but by 1982, they were nearly half. He wrote:

> Although employers deny that looks are important, students who are prepared to invest up to 400,000 yen (£1,100) reveal a better understanding of the psychology of interviews. They know when it comes to finding employment good looks count for more than good grades.

In America, where youth and conventional good looks are valued much more highly than in the UK, major structural alterations of the appearance are not confined to self-conscious youth or middle-aged women. The competition for jobs and promotion has forced many experienced middle-aged men executives into hospital for cosmetic surgery for fear of being passed over when it comes to promotion.

A leading New York plastic surgeon was quoted as saying in the early 1970s that the 'youth cult' was keeping him very busy, performing thousands of facelifts as well as other forms of self-improvement, often undertaken not by the bored housewife who feared her husband might run off with his secretary, but by career men and women who were determined not to be toppled off the ladder by younger, more attractive rivals.

Jim Jones, (not his real name), an advertising executive, reckons he saved his career by having a facelift whilst supposedly 'on vacation'. He was fed up with being passed over for promotions and overheard his boss remark how 'tired' he had been looking. In contrast, when he returned, to compliments all round about how 'rested' he looked, he was quickly promoted and then promoted again.

Every cosmetic surgeon in Britain can tell a handful of similar stories as well as others who 'saved' patients' marriages.

GETTING ADVICE

So, if the stigma of seeking cosmetic surgery is beginning to fade, how should you set about getting advice in the first place?

The obvious starting point is your GP.

But most GPs are untrained in cosmetic surgery and will be unaware of what can be done. On a list of priorities, they will probably also rate cosmetic surgery pretty low, and may tell you to go home

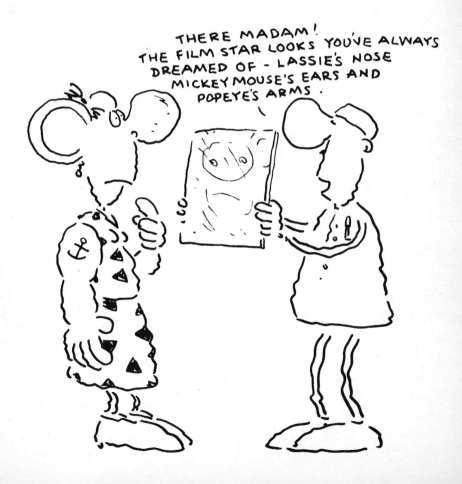

and forget about it. The role of the GP is to make sure there isn't some underlying organic or genetic disease which is curable *without* surgery.

But what if you can't forget about your problem? A good GP will give the matter further thought if he or she can see you are really bothered about it and should refer you to someone else, but not necessarily a plastic surgeon, for further counselling and advice. This person will try and find out whether cosmetic surgery will answer your problems. It might well be that your ears stick out, your chin recedes or your eyelids sag, but such defects may not be the cause of everything going wrong in your life.

The cause may have deeper psychological roots, which an expert will need to investigate, before booking you up to have your physical appearance altered. After all, there is no point in spending thousands of pounds on a non-essential operation if it does not achieve any worthwhile emotional results, even though some physical improvement may occur.

For example, if a middle-aged woman feels her husband is going to leave her for a younger woman, a facelift which makes her look ten years younger will make no difference if the marriage is dead and he is determined to end it.

The General Medical Council suggests that if your GP refuses to help you then you should consider asking for a second opinion, before answering an ad. If a second GP confirms the first's diagnosis, perhaps you are over-reacting to the supposed defect.

If, however, it is decided that cosmetic surgery is right for you, the GP should be able to refer you to a reputable cosmetic surgeon through a list—which is *not* available to the public or anyone non-medically qualified—which is provided by the British Association of Aesthetic Plastic Surgeons in London. This list states that the names on it are not the only cosmetic surgeons practising, but they will be definitely above board and above recrimination.

WARNING

Do not proceed with plastic surgery if you are not able to meet the surgeon for a proper consultation **before** the operation.

When you finally meet the cosmetic surgeon, usually for a nominal fee which is deducted from the final bill if you decide to go ahead, you will need to discuss carefully what you want to look like at the end, and whether this can actually be achieved. Yes, we'd all like to have eyes like Sophia Loren, or a nose like Julie Christie's, but can it ever be possible and would someone else's mouth suit *your* face?

A reputable cosmetic surgeon will look at the perceived physical abnormalty and tell the patient whether it can be improved upon. Leading cosmetic surgeons reckon they turn away at least one in ten would-be patients they see. One explained:

> It is either because, in all honesty, surgery would not improve anything, and despite what our critics say, we are definitely not touting for work— we don't need to—or because, after discussion, the patient can be reconciled to the defect, or because there are certain risks attached to the operation which make it impossible, no matter how desperate the patient might be.

You should not proceed with any operation which does not allow you to meet the surgeon until the day you go under the scalpel. Some clinics work on this basis, and invariably demand that you pay the bill in full before the appointed day. This is very bad practice because a direct consultation is a crucial part of the service.

WHAT RISKS ARE THERE IN COSMETIC SURGERY?

The risks vary according to the type of operation being considered, but the underlying mechanisms of bleeding, infection, compromised soft tissue circulation, and the formation of scars, are all quite similar. Added to this is the risk of anaesthesia itself.

Most side-effects are short-lived and any pain can be controlled with painkillers. After care is as important as the operation itself and, if neglected, can undermine any positive results. In 1984 a couple of cosmetic surgeons were struck off by the GMC because their after care procedure was very poor. (They were specializing in the removal of tattoos.)

THE COSMETIC SURGERY CLINIC ADS

Most people have seen the ads which offer a full range of cosmetic surgery, and may even have been tempted to make an appointment. If you write or telephone for details, you will usually be sent a booklet, which describes the operations in some detail, and which may, but usually does not, mention prices.

You are then invited to return a pre-paid form or card, booking an appointment, either with a non-medically-qualified counsellor, or with a cosmetic surgeon. If you choose the former, the consultation is usually free, and the counsellor may visit you in your home. If you decide to see the surgeon, there is usually what the clinic calls a 'modest charge', which will be around £20.

A well-known clinic close to Harley Street which specializes in cosmetic surgery, says in its introductory letter:

> We do realize you have an important decision to make and ideally we should like you to have the opportunity of visiting our clinic personally, and meeting one of our surgeons who will assess you for treatment and answer any questions you may have.
>
> However, we do appreciate this is not always possible and before deciding you may like an informal discussion at home with one of our female counsellors, who can give you a great deal of information on the treatment you require.

I telephoned the counsellor suggested by the clinic and pretended I was interested in having a nose operation. She correctly asked my age and, again correctly, told me that I was a suitable patient. She did not ask me how I felt about my nose, but proceeded to outline how and where the operation would be done and by whom. The surgeon, whom she named, had a long list of credentials and was 'the best', she said.

She warned against those doctors who had gone into cosmetic surgery who didn't know what they were doing but were just out to make a lot of money. She said the operation would cost a standard £1,650, and would include two nights in hospital and that they took Access and most credit cards to make payment easier. She was more enthusiastic about booking me up for a £20 consultation with the surgeon than seeing me herself, although she was willing to do so if I insisted. The consultation fee was deductible from the final bill.

Her whole emphasis was on selling the appointment and making the operation available—there were no waiting lists—rather than counselling, i.e. finding out what I looked like and whether the operation would be useful. I felt that had I taken it a step further, my commitment towards the idea would be that much firmer. More seriously, she did not mention my GP or ask whether I had seen him, or suggest that I should involve him at all.

The BMA and the GMC are as concerned about these people not consulting their doctors as they are about, the advertising of a doctor's services, since the medical profession has long insisted that its members refrain from self-advertisement. These ads do not print the surgeons' names, of course, but act as effectively as if they did, as far as the public are concerned.

I also contacted another well-known clinic near Heathrow, which advertises widely in newspapers and magazines. There I was told that I would definitely *not* have to consult or tell my GP about any proposed operation. Again, I was not queried about my motives, but they readily informed me that the basic charge for a nose job would be £1,250, for a one-night stay, and that the full amount would have to be paid before the operation. I could not choose my consultant but would be allocated to whoever was 'doing mornings or afternoons' on a random basis. I was not given their names but was assured they were 'properly qualified'.

Both the nature and profusion of cosmetic surgery ads themselves have outraged both the British Medical Association, which represents the country's 29,000 doctors, and the General Medical Council, the medical profession's disciplinary body.

The BMA's ruling council issued the following statement in 1981:

The Council of the BMA has discussed the direct access of patients to cosmetic surgery clinics. It deplores this practice and believes that the interests of the patients will be best served by referral through their general practitioner.

The Council further believes that doctors associated with such clinics should not consult with a patient in the absence of a letter of referral from the patient's personal or family doctor.

It added sternly: A doctor should not enter into a relationship with any clinic which does not follow the above procedure.

This policy remains today and although some doctors are angry because if they report any of their colleagues whom they believe to be flouting the rules of good medical practice, the General Medical Council can do nothing.

The current GMC guidelines suggest that a doctor who holds shares in an organization offering clinical services to the public should not work for it in a clinical capacity, nor should he or she allow his or her medical qualifications to form part of the advertising or descriptive literature.

Doctors who do not hold shares are allowed to work for such clinics providing it is on a regular sessional basis and not according to the number of patients they treat.

The GMC is currently revising its advisory guidelines on cosmetic clinic ads, and a spokesman said, 'We are aware of the problems and are very concerned to try to do something about it.' The hope is that the new guidelines will make it easier for the GMC to 'nail' the cowboy surgeons.

The GMC publishes a 'blue book' on professional conduct for doctors, and anyone thinking of taking action for negligence or unethical practice should consult this as a starter and then be prepared to back up a complaint with a declaration sworn in front of a JP.

Because of the various problems in the field, cosmetic surgeons themselves decided to form the British Association of Aesthetic Plastic Surgeons which has approximately 100 members, all of whom are qualified in either plastic surgery or some other medical speciality.

A spokesman for the British Association of Aesthetic Plastic Surgeons agreed that, ideally, the best way for a patient to approach a cosmetic surgeon was through his or her own GP. But this was not always practical, he said, and anyway many GPs would rather their patients just answered an ad and dealt with the matter themselves.

The difficulty is how *do* you find a reputable cosmetic surgeon *without* going through a GP or answering an ad?

The aesthetic surgeons' association has found the present rules difficult and is currently campaigning for a system under which it could release the names and addresses of member cosmetic surgeons to the public. Would-be patients could then read down the list and pick out a few names—probably locally—and make inquiries from there.

Mr Peter Davis a consultant at St Thomas's and Westminster Hospitals in London told a conference of plastic surgeons organized by BAAPS in 1988, that because the public is faced with an 'information vacuum', individuals are being driven into the minefield of the private clinics where it is impossible for them to differentiate between bonafide practices and the less reputable ones. Mr Davis, secretary of BAAPS, says:

At these places patients may not see the surgeon until an hour before their operation. They may have to pay cash in advance and there is no guarantee the surgeon has any training in plastic surgery. To members of the public we are like a secret society

Meanwhile, remember the old maxim, 'Let the buyer beware.' Lastly, do not be too swayed by the 'before' and 'after' photographs. Rather like those in the slimming ads, the 'before' pictures are often taken in a deliberately unflattering light/angle etc, whilst the latter are given the reverse treatment.

The particular clinics I spoke to are reputable, but always check carefully—there are many dubious ones.

THE MOST COMMON OPERATIONS AND THEIR POSSIBLE SIDE-EFFECTS

The first thing to note about all cosmetic surgery is that some sort of scarring is inevitable. However, this can be minimized by the surgeon who should make sure that facelifts scars, for example, appear just behind the hairline. Male facelifts are planned so they do not interfere with beards or sideburns because, even if the patient sports a beard now, his tastes may change later on and he would not want to be stuck with either a beard or a nasty scar. Nose and ear operations can usually be done in such a way that the scars form part of the natural lines already on the patient's face.

Meticulous care in surgical wound closures should ensure the best 'finish' possible, but it is impossible to predict the final outcome of surgery for a minimum of six months and probably not for a year or even longer.

Patients are expected to adhere strictly to the recommended post-operative care and this may include the regular application of dressings as well as some restriction in activities, plus of course follow-up visits. It is therefore important to be able to get to your chosen surgeon reasonably easily.

FACELIFT

A facelift or rhytidectomy is any operation involving various procedures which raise the facial skin and reduce hanging folds or 'lines'. Facelifts normally involve the skin of the neck, the region under the chin, the cheeks and the temples. The forehead and eyelids may be included in a facelift, but they are normally done separately. Indeed, often a patient seeking a facelift will be offered the alternative blepharoplasty (eyelid surgery) if the ageing is concentrated (as it often is) around the eyes.

Once removed, the fatty tissue 'bags' usually do not return.

The going rate for a full facelift in London is between £1,500 and £2,000, depending on who performs the operation and where. The results last for only four to eight years.

ALTERNATIVES TO FACELIFTS

Although the manufacturers of hundreds of different 'magic potions' claim otherwise, the facelift is the only way yet devised to actually make the face look younger. Cosmetics can improve the surface of the skin, but the actual structure below can only be altered for the better by surgical scalpel. Similarly, so-called chin supports or facial muscle exercises are pointless and may even, in some circumstances, be harmful. For example, constant vibration massage may result in more rapid shrinkage of the underlying delicate fatty tissue and produce the opposite effect to that which is being sought.

There is, alas, no substitute for the facelift if the facial skin sags heavily and the underlying skin muscle is poor. Most people put up with the signs of ageing as inevitable and unavoidable, but others, (mostly the rich, and people in the theatre and on televisions), regard a facelift as an absolute essential —which may be delayed, but not avoided altogether.

As the skin on the face ages, the fatty tissue lining just under the skin shrinks, causing the outer skin, the bit we see, to fit more loosely, and eventually sag into folds. On top of all this, the various contours of the face become more evident where the facial muscles attach to the under surface of the skin. The resulting folds of skin become more prominent from a combination of muscular action and the force of gravity.

The most dramatic physical changes occur under the chin (the so-called double-chin) and around the jowl and near the corners of the eyebrows (the so-called 'crow's-feet' or laughter lines) and mouth, where the face has creased into a million smiles and frowns over the years.

These changes often tend to accentuate the shape of the nose, which becomes sharper in relation to the rest of the face and any imperfections here become more noticeable as the overlying soft tissues are reduced in volume. The area around the dental ridge can often appear 'tighter' because of shrinkage and, these all conspire to make the overall appearance unattractive.

Those with red or blonde hair tend to age faster as do those with dry or thin skin. Over-exposure to the sun over a number of years will age the skin substantially faster (see chapter nine).

The facelift operation is tailor-made to suit the patient, according to his or her features and where the skin has aged fastest. The basic operation is designed to lift, stretch and remove sagging skin whilst supporting the underlying facial muscles.

The ideal age for a facelift is the early 40s, for although the operations can be performed in the 60s and 70s, the more overstretched the muscles are, the harder the operations become.

FACELIFT AFTERCARE

Patients are usually advised not to exercise the muscles of the face too strenuously, and avoid talking, laughing or chewing vigorously. This could produce pressure which would cause bleeding and undermine the final results of the operation. A facelift is a long and major operation and patients are advised to take at least a fortnight off work afterwards. they can go out, but have to cover up their scars and bruising.

POSSIBLE SIDE-EFFECTS

Sometimes, although not usually, there may be some limited blood collection under the skin and if this is heavy, the surgeon may need to re-open an incision to remove the clotted blood.

There may be some temporary lag in the normal motion of facial muscles as well as a feeling of numbness and tension in the neck and cheek areas as well as around the ear. There is also some bruising and swelling which can last two weeks.

Some further sagging can occur even after six months and a secondary operation may be necessary. This does not mean the surgeon was incompetent—it's just that the results cannot be accurately predicted beforehand. No other side-effects have been noted and all those listed above should be of limited duration, i.e. patients should not worry about the possibility of constant check-ups to make sure their incisions are not breaking out or the blood clotting up underneath!

There are several additional surgical techniques that can be carried out, either with a facelift, or separately. These include chemosurgery (not to be confused with chemotherapy, the drug treatment used on cancer patients), otherwise known as a 'face-peel', or dermabrasion, or collagen implants.

CHEMOSURGERY OR FACE PEEL

THE PROCEDURE

This is a relatively new operation which uses powerful chemicals to literally destroy, by burning off, the outer (dead) layers of the skin. By doing this, it lays bare a deep layer from which the new skin can grow. The operation sounds and looks horrific and to me is definitely not the sort of thing anyone sane would want to inflict on themselves from choice, never mind paying £1,000 or more for the privilege!

One seasoned former beauty editor of one of the top glossies was recently shown around one of the Harley Street clinics which advertises these operations and was appalled by what she was shown. Ladies with burned faces made her remark in horror, 'If we found that they were doing that to people in prisons there would be an international outcry and Britain would be reported to Amnesty International for torture of the most horrific kind!'

Christopher Margrave, in his book *Cosmetic Surgery: Facing the Facts* (Penguin, 1985) comments:

A full and effective peel cannot be achieved without pain, discomfort and without inconvenience or without the patient looking horrific for a few days. However, by the time the new skin has matured, the finer lines will have disappeared and even deeper grooves will have become less obvious.

The treatment, according to him and others, is ideal for the fair-skinned patient whose skin has aged prematurely with many fine wrinkles, probably from years of excessive sunbathing. Since the process bleaches the skin, it is not suitable for darker skins.

The face is normally peeled without a full anaesthetic, which, again, sounds horrific, but any patients who are nervous can be given one. The skin is first cleansed and then smeared with a cotton bud dipped in a caustic mixture containing phenol and crotol oil. This is done until the surface of the skin has turned white. There is usually a stinging pain which is controlled by drugs and the skin is then sealed with adhesive tape and the patient put to rest for two days. The process is essentially no different from what takes place in second-degree burns.

After two days, the adhesive is removed, again with the help of painkillers, and the top dead layers which have literally been burned off, are peeled away attached to the sticky tape. During the two days, the eyes and the mouth tissues swell dramatically and eating, drinking and talking become very difficult.

The newly-exposed tender skin underneath is coated with antiseptic powder

---

WARNING

It is possible that a chemical peel can result in a skin **permanently** sensitive to the sun.
In a few cases, deaths have followed a chemical peel.

which forms a caked crust. The swellings gradually subside, the eyelids open and eating and drinking become less of a problem.

On the fifth or sixth day, the crust is softened with cold cream or vaseline and gently removed with the aid of soap and lukewarm water.

CHEMICAL PEEL— AFTERCARE

The newly-formed skin, which the body has naturally produced, will be light pink and looked scorched as if sunburned and will be abnormally sensitive. It has to be kept moist with creams or it will dry out and crack. After two weeks, the patient can wear light make-up to disguise the paler colour which lasts up to three weeks before assuming a normal skin shade.

POSSIBLE SIDE-EFFECTS

The patient has to avoid sunlight for a further two months otherwise the skin can discolour. The skin anyway will be very sensitive to the sun during this phase and a cream with a suncreen (UV filter) is essential. I know of one woman who has undergone this operation who says she can never go out in the sun because her face starts burning immediately. Given that there is a likelihood that most patients seeking this type of operation have already damaged their skins by excessive sun-exposure, it seems only fair that future patients are warned about this possibility. Unfortunately, like most people who are dissatisfied with cosmetic surgery operations, she has not complained so her experience is not being passed on to the clinic concerned.

Multiple white spots can appear after a couple of weeks, signifying blockage of the sebaceous glands. This can be remedied by lightly rubbing the affected area with soap and water.

More serious, but rarer, is that if an area has been burnt too deeply, the skin will heal not by forming a nice new layer but by scarring and even distorting the adjacent structures such as the eyelids or lips. These scars have then to be treated as scars sustained in accidents, with further surgery.

THE ULTIMATE 'SIDE-EFFECT'

Finally, if you are still thinking of a chemical peel, you should know that in *Unwanted Effects of Cosmetics and Durgs Used in Dermatology* (Elsevier, 1985), the Dutch dermatologists J. P. Nater and A. C. de Groot, note that several deaths have occurred in individuals following face-peels. They suggest that the process is not risky as long as the phenol is applied slowly, over at least an hour, and as long as the dose is carefully monitored and kept below the fatal level estimated to be in excess of eight grams. They note that where death has occurred, this has taken place within 24 hours, so there is no need to worry if you have already undergone this 'treatment'.

COLLAGEN IMPLANTS

These are relatively new—although collagen has been around for some time as a 'magic' ingredient in many of the more expensive skin creams, where it is of dubious value.

However, collagen as a prepared injectable substance does appear to work by combining with normal tissues—which also contain collagen—to fill out small skin depressions without the use of surgery. The collagen injections can be used to puff out deep wrinkle lines as well as old scars from injuries, or pock-marks left over from chicken-pox. The treatment is virtually painless as the injection contains anaesthetic. However it is expensive—several sessions are required to get the right results. The treatment is also not as permanent as a full facelift and top-ups will be required as part of a maintenance programme.

Costs vary, depending on how much you have to have done. One injection plus consultations, etc. could cost as little as £100, but a full course can cost £500 or more.

NOSE REFINEMENT (RHINOPLASTY)

Rhinoplasty is one of the most common types of cosmetic surgery. Many people don't like the shape of the nose they were born with. Nature can play some cruel tricks with this feature.

Because the nose continues to change shape up to the age of about twenty, the first question a reputable clinic should ask any enquirer is 'How old are you?' Children can be operated upon, depending on the degree of disfigurement, their emotional attitude and overall physical development. Any clinic which automatically says it will operate on a young child regardless of these other factors should be treated with caution. There is no upper age limit to this form of surgery.

Changes in the nasal contour are made by altering the underlying structure of bone and cartilage. The skin is then draped or moulded over the new base to achieve the desired result. The operation is performed inside the nose and so leaves no external scars.

The cost quoted for this operation by the Mediform Clinic was £1,650, regardless of age or any personal details about the patient, and would involve two nights spent in a private hospital. Unlike most cosmetic surgery, rhinoplasty can sometimes be carried out on the NHS, especially if the nose was misshapen in an accident rather than at birth and if it gives rise to breathing problems.

AFTER THE OPERATION

The patient has to wear a cast for 10 days to protect the new nose from injury. Nasal swelling and bruising remain for up to two weeks, but final settlement and softening will take up to nine months, so there is a long time to wait before the final results can be properly appreciated.

As with facelifts, final results cannot be predicted accurately and some patients will be disappointed with the outcome, especially if their expectations have been unrealistic. Each operation is different and, although photographs can give an indication of what can be achieved, the end result, and one's reaction to it, is highly individual.

EAR CORRECTION (OTOPLASTY)

Has Prince Charles had his ears fixed or not? No-one knows, and probably we'll never find out, but everyone remembers how, as a small boy and young man, his ears used to be much more prominent than they are now.

He was not alone. Children, especially boys (whose ears are usually more noticeable because of the way their hair is cut), are teased mercilessly at school if they have unusually large or protruding ears.

So much so, that 90 per cent of all surgery on prominent ears is carried out on children. They have to be at least six, by which time the ear has stopped growing; if operated on before, normal growth will be impaired. Any clinic prepared to operate on children younger than six should be avoided. The operation is usually done on an out-patient basis. It is carried out under a local anaesthetic and is painless. For these reasons, it is a relatively inexpensive operation.

242

AFTERCARE

A large protective head bandage is worn for about ten days and the swelling will take four weeks to subside, so the initial results can be disappointing unless the patient is properly forewarned.

If there is any persistent pain afterwards, an infection may have occurred and it is important that this is treated swiftly because, if it involved the framework of the ear, part of the cartilage may be destroyed, leaving a permanent deformity. A common side-effect is the appearance of a small ulcer—the result of pressure when the ears have been slept on—and this usually heals itself.

Scars are hidden behind the ear so they are very difficult to see.

CHIN SURGERY (MENTOPLASTY)

The underdeveloped or receding chin can be a source of misery for the owner. A cosmetic operation involves the use of silicone implants, as used in breast surgery, and these can be shaped according to the wishes of the patient.

Sometimes, an underdeveloped chin is associated with nasal deformity and a chin operation alone will not result in an overall balanced appearance of the patient's face. Some patients undergoing a nose operation also have to have their chins altered at the same time. Similarly, an overdeveloped or protruding chin may be related to a dental deformity which has to be studied if surgical treatment is being considered. An operation to correct an abnormally shaped chin will therefore have to take careful note of either the nose or the jaw and teeth of the patient.

Surgery of the lower jaw is complicated because this is the area which houses the single nerve serving the lower teeth, the sides of the tongue, the chin and all the bone and soft tissues around the lower half of the mouth.

HIGH CHEEK BONES

High cheek bones are generally what distinguishes the exquisitely beautiful males and females from the rest of the human race. Lovely eyes, pretty noses and attractive sexy lips all help, but it is the actual shape of the face which distinguishes a beautiful woman or handsome man from someone who is merely 'attractive'.

Cosmetic surgeons can create high cheek bones by inserting custom-designed silicone implants into pockets created under the skin just over the cheek bones with a cut made either high inside the mouth or just in front of the ear. The results can be dramatically effective, but they depend on the rest of the facial features being good and well-balanced.

The potential risks of silicone implants are the same in the cheek as anywhere else in the body. Silicone is synthetic and biologically inert and is easily sterilized. It can be made as soft and squidgy or hard and muscular as desired, depending on whether it is being implanted in the nose, chin, cheeks, or breasts.

BREAST SURGERY (MAMMAPLASTY)

Breast surgery can involve augmentation, reduction or reconstruction and can be useful for women who are genuinely disturbed by defects in their breasts and surgery is rarely performed before they are mature—the age of 18 at least. For older women, because the breast is involved in milk production during pregnancy, careful consideration has to be given to the rest of their state of health and lifestyle. Many patients seek the help of a cosmetic surgeon if their formerly firm breasts have sagged after childbirth. Others sometimes do so because substantial weight-loss has led to sagging breasts.

Breast surgery can also be used for women who have had a breast partially removed because of breast cancer—in which case the history of the disease must be very carefully checked. For this type of operation, the involvement of your GP and/or hospital consultant is essential. If you have a history of breast abnormality, do not consider cosmetic surgery of the breast with any surgeon who is willing to bypass your GP.

Breast enlargement—or uplift, which is a more appropriate term—is one of the two most common cosmetic operations—the other being facelifts—carried out in the world. In America, more than 30,000 women a year have their breasts surgically enlarged, and today more than half a million women are walking round with artificially enlarged breasts.

WARNING

If you have had breast surgery because of cancer, your GP and/or consultant **must** be consulted about any subsequent cosmetic surgery of the breasts.

Surgeons use synthetic silicone either as a solid material—a 'prosthesis', which has been described as looking like 'a stranded jellyfish'—or as an inflatable silicone bag. The latter has the advantage that it can be inserted through a very small hole in its collapsed state, leaving only a tiny scar. This method is therefore increasingly popular.

Silicone in its injected soft oily form should never be used to increase the size of the breast because the complications in terms of pain, infection, ulceration, displacement and distortion can be appalling. Under no circumstances even consider this type of breast enlargement.

Any surgery on the breast can, and probably will, adversely affect any erotic stimulation a woman has hitherto enjoyed, and this should be pointed out by the surgeon or counselling staff, in case it is important to the patient. It should also be realized that an enlarged breast does not behave exactly like a normal breast. If you are lying on your back on the beach, your new breasts will point skyward—while, all about you, unimproved breasts flatten out under the force of gravity.

RISKS AND SIDE-EFFECTS

Despite many rumours to the contrary, there has never been any demonstrated risk between the silicone prosthesis and future development of breast cancer. However, one report in 1980 did find four cases in which breast cancer had been detected in women who had undergone silicone implants for cosmetic purposes. Future diagnosis of 'lumps and bumps' can also be made more complicated if a woman has had her breasts enlarged surgically.

WARNING

Breast enlargement should **never** be done with injected soft silicone.

You should always remind your doctor that you have undergone mammaplasty when you have a breast examination, and tell your family planning counsellor so that she can prescribe the most appropriate form of pill.

The implants should not interfere with breast-feeding if a woman subsequently becomes pregnant. Indeed, most women forget they have had their breasts operated on after the first couple of months. But in about 15 per cent of operations, the breast may become more firm because of the tightening of the fibrous capsule which forms around the implant. A good surgeon should move the implant around a bit to prevent this occurring, but a second surgical re-opening may be necessary.

BREAST REDUCTION

Overlarge breasts can cause as many psychological problems as undersized or sagging ones, and because the reducing of them is a major operation and often involves the nipples too, it is usually more expensive than enlargement.

Costs vary, but any operation which requires a private hospital bed for two or three days will cost at least £1,000 and probably considerably more. It is possible to find surgeons who will operate for less than £500 on an out-patient patient or overnight basis but make sure any one offering a cut-price service is doing a proper job.

WARNING
If you want to breast feed, do not consider surgery for breast reduction.

RISKS AND SIDE-EFFECTS

Unlike breast enlargement, reduction will normally mean that breast-feeding will not be possible in future. If this is an important consideration, then the operation is not recommended, i.e. if the woman has not had, and expects to have children and might want to breast-feed them.

Ten per cent of patients experience a strange complication called fat necrosis, which is caused by disturbance of the blood supply within the breasts as they are being 're-designed'. This manifests itself as small hard lumps which eventually heal themselves, but which meanwhile can make the patient panic, thinking, wrongly, that she has developed breast cancer.

There may be considerable scarring, but this is usually preferable for the woman who has suffered from unmanageable breasts.

BREAST SURGERY IN MEN

A small number of men *do* undergo surgery to remove breasts which have over-developed as a result of hormonal upset or because of kidney disease or as a side-effect of some drugs.

This is much more common among boys at puberty, of whom *one in three* have some degree of breast enlargement. In most cases, their breasts return to their normal size in about 18 months, but some do not, and the boys either learn to live with their shape or suffer what they regard as an effeminate 'deformity'.

CHAPTER NINETEEN

CONCLUSIONS

So, where does all of this leave us? There is no reason why you should want to give up using cosmetics, perfume, or toiletries after reading this book.

However, you might now begin to change your shopping habits and wonder why you have wasted so much money on those anti-wrinkle creams and revert to the cheaper, simpler moisturizers. You may also decide to stick with semi-permanent hair dyes, or even your natural hair colour and shape, instead of repeatedly applying all those chemicals to your head.

On a more profound social level, if you're not already aware of the fact that it is possible to buy a wide range of products which have not been tested on animals (nor those which contain animal extracts) you might like to switch your brand. Similarly, if you've never thought about the consequences of using aerosols such as hairsprays and anti-perspirants, I hope you will think about the conservation and health issues.

Like all such acts, including voting in elections, the individual gesture does not seem to count for much, but thousands, or millions, of individuals doing the same thing obviously make a great impact, not only on an industry, but in the wider world. The cosmetics industry has, after all, been forced to change its policy on aerosols, for example.

Of course, fashion influences the amount we spend on certain types of cosmetics—currently for example, the expenditure on hair-styling products is booming, whilst the sums spent on perfumes is pretty much the same as it has been for the last five years, and sales of talcum powders and hand lotions are in decline.

The heavily made-up look has been out of fashion for about 20 years now. So, women are now using less foundation and face make-up. However, the actual value of the overall sales have risen by 10 per cent during the 1980s and we now spend £70 million a year on such products.

Similarly, although false eyelashes and the dark-ringed eyes of the '60s are no longer fashionable, we spend nearly £100 million a year simply on keeping those eyelashes fluttering and those eyes alluring. Despite the fact that the vast majority of women work, and don't have the time or the lifestyle to brandish immaculate fingernails, collectively we spend £43 million a year simply on our nails.

Add to the make-up the vast sums spent on beauty and grooming gadgets— £111 million on shaving gear, £26.5 million on hairdryers, and you can see it is a vast industry.

We now spend over £800 million a year on cosmetics, toiletries and perfumes, and that sum rises every year. As a nation we spend more in the chemist's shop buying cosmetics and toiletries and home treatments than we do on all insurance, or all books, newspapers and magazines. We only spent fractionally more on our postal and telephone bills. We even spend more on cosmetics than we do on our national tipple—tea— (£600 million)—though not, of course, as much as we spend on booze.

There are no signs that, as a whole, younger people are using fewer cosmetics than their parents' generation, although of course, many individuals shun it altogether. The big difference is that boys are using more cosmetics than ever before and often have drawers full of stuff their mothers (let alone their fathers) might be embarrassed to use.

I have been careful to steer clear of the vast subject of dieting in this book, simply because it would be in danger of swamping everything else. But of course, the cosmetics industry has more than a passing interest in our shape and weight, as opposed to our facial appearance. There is a whole industry making creams supposed to firm up the bust or thighs, and of course the sun-tan lotion business relies on persuading us all to want to look pretty sexy in as few clothes as possible.

A survey carried out by *Diet and Lifestyle* magazine in 1987 found that at least 50 per cent of the 1,000 women interviewed reckoned their figures were what attracted them to men in the first place.

A third of the women had considered cosmetic surgery because they were not satisfied that even the most skilful use of cosmetics and perfumes could improve on what nature had given them at birth and what they had done to themselves since! Is this a failure of the industry to come up with the goods— literally—or a measure of people's insecurity in the mating stakes?

I am inclined to think the latter, and that the models who have been turned into international celebrities have set standards that every schoolgirl longs to emulate. The industry, through its ads, seeks to make us believe this is possible—if only we can find the right lipstick, the best blusher, the most nourishing skin cream and the most sexy perfume, and so on.

So what's wrong with that? Does it really matter that women set themselves such impossible goals, and make themselves miserable if they fail to reach them? The feminists would argue that it is, because dwelling on physical appearance undermines other qualities, which may be substantial. Yet increasingly men too are falling into this 'beauty trap'.

My own feeling is that it is sad that some women, especially teenagers and those who feel unhappy about growing older, get things out of proportion. For some, having their nose fixed, or their crow's feet removed, is a stepping stone to winning a gorgeous man, bringing back their roaming husbands, or restoring a flagging sex-life. Sadly, these things rarely work, but if the individual feels better afterwards, then no harm has been done.

However, if the expectations have been unrealistic and they are disappointed, then the psychological damage can be enormous. This is really the bone I have to pick with the industry, and in particular the beauty ads and 'advertorials', along with the sweet-talking sales-assistants whose only interest is to sell, sell, sell.

On the other hand, there is no doubt that a new hairstyle, a lavish spray of expensive perfume, or a luxurious facial can all do their bit to enhance people's self-esteem and that can be reflected impressively in the way they behave either at work or at home, or socially.

Men and women from all walks of life admit to feelings of insecurity about their looks and, as a consequence, place enormous trust and expectation in their hairdressers and other beauty professionals. In a recent BBC documentary about hairdressing, Vidal Sassoon and other hairdressers told how a haircut could 'make or break' a customer's life for the next day, weekend, or even the next three months. This is a power the dentist, doctor or teacher rarely wields.

If you read the beauty books written by the world's beauties, you will find that they all stress that beauty to a large extent comes from *inside*. They can afford to express such soothing sentiments when they know that they have got almost perfect features, bone structure, complexion, figure, etc., plus a host of professional beauticians to enhance it all and a bottomless bank balance to pay for it.

What is interesting is that older women are now recognized as sexy and attractive, despite their advancing years. Joanna Lumley, Catherine Deneuve, Linda Evans, Jane Fonda, Sophia Loren and a host of other 'middle-aged' beauties have now ensured that women do not need to start searching for the anti-ageing creams and cosmetic surgeon's scalpel in their late 30s.

Not long ago, such actresses would have been relegated to playing grandmothers once they had passed the age of 30 or so. Now, the stars of *Dallas* and *Dynasty* are playing at being sex kittens in their fifties.

Meanwhile, singers like Cher, Sandie Shaw, and Tina Turner demonstrate that, even in the youth-orientated pop business, women can survive as long as the eternally youthful Cliff Richard.

Who knows, if the trend continues, we may all be actively seeking formulas to 'age' ourselves from puberty onwards—and painting in crow's feet to suggest that we have already 'lived'! There would be nothing particularly weird about this—after all, the Elizabethans painted veins on their foreheads to denote their blue-bloodedness! And the Chinese revere old age.

One thing is sure, everything in beauty has its day and fashions and fads will return. Nothing is new, despite the claims made for each 'innovation' launched by the industry. Today's merchants of anti-ageing formulas invoke 'space-age' technology but cell-therapy has been around for a log time. Back in the 1920s people were injecting themselves with monkey gland extracts and before that fresh tissue from dog's testicles was said to be a marvellous rejuvenator of skin and muscle. And to think some of us might feel squeamish about using placenta from sheep!

Nor are the consumer complaints about the claims made for such anti-ageing formulas new. A search of newspaper cuttings in American archives retrieved a 1958 clipping which criticized the anti-ageing claims made for Helena Rubenstein's *Beauty for Life Capsules.*

The product, containing vitamins, Royal Jelly and gelatin, was claimed to also 'ease heart disease, muscular dystrophy and many other disorders'. Not surprisingly, the ad had to be changed.

Thirty years on, the Food and Drug Administration is still battling with the cosmetics companies to stop them making unsubstantiated claims about their products. No doubt in 30 years' time, they will still be at it.

Unless, and this seems unlikely, men and women, worldwide, decide that they are happy with what nature intended and that there is no need for pills, potions, and magic, and dreams in bottles, phials and spray-cans, the cosmetics and beauty industry will continue to boom.

My hope is that the obsession that many women have about beauty, and their (often quite hopeless) personal quest for it, will wane. Perhaps as men and women become more equal all over the world and more men experience the insecurity and misery of the 'beauty trap' then they will cease to judge women quite so much by looks alone.

I take comfort from the fact that only three people in my life have ever presumed to admonish me for not taking greater care of my appearance. All of them were men. The first was a balding and particularly ugly elderly colleague who felt I should wear shorter skirts, sexy black tights and lots of lipstick, to look 'feminine' and decorative around the office.

The second was menopausal and depressed and felt I should dress and make-up more and flirt to cheer him up at work. The third, a millionaire playboy declared that he felt I was not 'glossy' enough to be his constant social companion (I had not actually applied for the role). Several weeks later he telephoned and told me his stunning news—he had fallen in love with a girl who not only rarely wore make-up, but also like me, horror of horrors, bit her nails!

There's hope for us all yet!

INDEX